Dx/Rx: Leukemia

John M. Burke, MD

Rocky Mountain Cancer Centers
Colorado Springs, CO

Series Editor: Manish A. Shah, MD

JONES AND BARTLETT PUBLISHERS

Sudbury, Massachusetts

BOSTON TORONTO LONDON SINGAPORE

World Headquarters
Jones and Bartlett Publishers
40 Tall Pine Drive
Sudbury, MA 01776
978-443-5000
info@jbpub.com
www.jbpub.com

Jones and Bartlett Publishers Canada
6339 Ormindale Way
Mississauga, Ontario L5V 1J2
CANADA

Jones and Bartlett Publishers International
Barb House, Barb Mews
London W6 7PA
UK

Jones and Bartlett's books and products are available through most bookstores and online booksellers. To contact Jones and Bartlett Publishers directly, call 800-832-0034, fax 978-443-8000, or visit our website, www.jbpub.com.

Substantial discounts on bulk quantities of Jones and Bartlett's publications are available to corporations, professional associations, and other qualified organizations. For details and specific discount information, contact the special sales department at Jones and Bartlett via the above contact information or send an email to specialsales@jbpub.com.

Library of Congress Cataloging-in-Publication Data
Burke, John (John McEvoy), 1970-
Dx/Rx. Leukemia / by John Burke.
p. ; cm.
Includes bibliographical references.
ISBN 0-7637-2738-5
1. Leukemia—Handbooks, manuals, etc. I. Title. II. Title: Leukemia.
[DNLM: 1. Leukemia—Handbooks. WH 39 B959d 2005]
RC643.B85 2005
616.99′419—dc22

2005024329

Production Credits
Executive Publisher: Christopher Davis
Associate Editor: Kathy Richardson
Production Director: Amy Rose
Production Editor: Renée Sekerak
Production Assistant: Rachel Rossi
Associate Marketing Manager: Laura Kavigian
Manufacturing Buyer: Therese Connell
Cover Design: Anne Spencer
Photo Research: Kimberly Potvin
Composition: ATLIS Graphics
Printing and Binding: Malloy, Inc.
Cover Printing: Malloy, Inc.

Printed in the United States of America
09 08 07 06 05 10 9 8 7 6 5 4 3 2 1

Contents

Editor's Preface

Welcome to the Dx/Rx Oncology series. This is a new series of handbooks focusing on the practical management of common malignancies. The current book, *Dx/Rx: Leukemia,* is a comprehensive, yet succinct, overview of acute and chronic leukemia, the myelodysplastic syndromes and plasma cell dyscrasias. Although these malignancies are relatively uncommon, their diagnoses and appropriate management are essential for the practicing oncologist. Dr. Burke does an excellent job organizing the handbook in a natural, easy to understand flow—critical for the complex management of a patient with a bone marrow derived malignancy. I believe you will find this handbook, and the entire handbook series, an invaluable resource to you and your colleagues.

Manish A. Shah

CHAPTER 1

General Features of Acute Leukemias

Introduction

- The two primary categories of acute leukemia are acute myeloid (or myelogenous) leukemia (AML) and acute lymphoblastic (or lymphocytic) leukemia (ALL).
- The clinical features, diagnostic evaluation, and supportive treatments for both types of acute leukemia are similar and are discussed in this chapter.
- Details about other aspects of these diseases, including epidemiology, risk factors, classification, genetics, and therapies, are discussed in Chapters 2 (AML) and 4 (ALL).

Definition of Acute Leukemias

- Acute leukemias are clonal, neoplastic proliferations of immature hematopoietic cells in the bone marrow and blood. This process results in the accumulation of these immature hematopoietic cells, or blasts, in the bone marrow and in failure of these same cells to differentiate into normal, mature blood cells.
- In 1976, a group of hematopathologists formed the French-American-British (FAB) Cooperative Group in order to establish a widely accepted definition and classification of acute leukemias.[1] Subsequently, the group revised its classification of acute leukemias as new diagnostic techniques became available.[2-4] In general, according to FAB criteria, the diagnosis of acute leukemia requires that at least 30% of the nucleated cells in the bone marrow be blasts.
- In 2001, the World Health Organization (WHO) proposed a new classification scheme for leukemias and other hematologic malignancies.[5] According to the

WHO, the diagnosis of AML now requires that only 20% of the nucleated cells in the bone marrow be myeloid blasts. The rationale behind this modification is that outcomes in patients with 20–30% myeloid blasts may be similar to those in patients with greater than 30% blasts.[6,7]

Clinical Features of Acute Leukemias

- Symptoms
  - Anemia may cause fatigue, dyspnea with exertion, and congestive heart failure.
  - Leukopenia may result in fevers and infections.
  - Thrombocytopenia may cause bruising and bleeding from other sites.
  - Bone pain may occur, most commonly in children with ALL.
  - If present, a mediastinal mass (more common in ALL) may produce cough, dyspnea, and chest pain.
  - Leukemia involving the central nervous system (CNS) may cause cranial neuropathies, most commonly involving the sixth and seventh cranial nerves; headaches; and nausea or vomiting. CNS leukemia is more common in ALL than in AML.
- Signs
  - Anemia may cause pallor.
  - Thrombocytopenia may cause petechiae, ecchymoses, and retinal hemorrhages.
  - Hepatomegaly, splenomegaly, and lymphadenopathy occur more commonly in ALL than in AML.
  - Infiltration of gums may cause gingival hypertrophy, particularly in acute monocytic leukemia.
  - Infiltration of skin may cause a rash, called "leukemia cutis."
  - CNS leukemia may cause papilledema.
  - Rarely, a solid mass of myeloid leukemia cells, called "granulocytic sarcoma," can involve any organ, including the skin, bones, and breast.
  - Leukostasis due to a markedly elevated white blood cell (WBC) count may cause hypoxia and dyspnea, particularly in AML.

- Laboratory features
  - The WBC count may be low, normal, or elevated. Markedly elevated WBC counts (ie, >100,000/μL) are characteristic of T-cell ALL or acute monocytic leukemia.
  - Neutropenia, anemia, and thrombocytopenia are usually present.
  - Although renal function is usually not affected, occasionally tumor lysis syndrome exists at presentation, causing hyperkalemia, hyperphosphatemia, an elevated lactate dehydrogenase (LDH) level, an elevated uric acid level, and renal insufficiency.
  - Acute promyelocytic leukemia often causes disseminated intravascular coagulopathy, characterized by prolongation of the prothrombin and partial thromboplastin times, diminished fibrinogen levels, and a bleeding tendency.

Diagnostic Evaluation

- History and physical exam
- Blood tests, including a complete blood count (CBC), peripheral blood smear, chemistry panel, LDH, uric acid, prothrombin time (PT), activated partial thromboplastin time (PTT), fibrinogen, and blood type
- Typing of human leukocyte antigens (HLA typing) should be performed at the time of diagnosis in patients who might be considered for allogeneic hematopoietic cell transplantation (usually patients under age 55 years, although HLA typing can also be performed in patients over age 55 years if nonmyeloablative hematopoietic cell transplantation on an investigational protocol can be considered). Siblings should also undergo HLA typing.
- Bone marrow aspirate and biopsy
  - A myeloperoxidase stain is generally performed to help distinguish between AML and ALL.
  - Immunophenotyping
    - Antigen groups called "clusters of differentiation" (CDs) can be identified on the surface of hematopoietic cells by monoclonal antibodies directed at those CDs.

  - Certain antigens correlate with cell lineage (called "lineage-associated antigens"), and a few antigens are considered to be specific for a certain lineage (called "lineage-specific antigens"). Table 1-1 lists some CDs and their associated lineages.[8,9]
  - Immunophenotyping by flow cytometry should be performed in all newly diagnosed patients with acute leukemia. The main purposes of immunophenotyping are to help distinguish AML from ALL, to identify biphenotypic leukemias, to help distinguish between different subtypes of both AML and ALL, and to help monitor for minimal residual disease.
- Genetic testing
  - Conventional cytogenetic analysis
    - Clonal cytogenetic abnormalities can be detected in the majority of patients with AML or ALL. These cytogenetic abnormalities are often

Table 1-1: Selected Clusters of Differentiation Antigens and Their Associated Cell Lineages

Cell lineage	Antigens
Lymphoid B	CD19, CD20, cytoplasmic CD22,* CD23, CD79a*
Lymphoid T	CD1, CD2, cytoplasmic CD3,* CD4, CD5, CD7, CD8
Myelomonocytic	Myeloperoxidase,* CD11c, CD13, CD33, CD117 (c-kit)
Megakaryocytic	CD41, CD61
Erythrocytic	Glycophorin A
NK cells	CD16, CD56
Non-lineage-specific	TdT, HLA-DR

*Considered lineage-specific.

HLA, human leukocyte antigen.

important in the pathogenesis of the disease, serve as prognostic markers, and influence treatment decisions.
- Conventional cytogenetic analysis involves the examination of chromosomes in early metaphase, when the chromosome structure is best defined. The chromosomes of approximately 20 cells are studied for mutations, including deletions, additions, and translocations.
- Cytogenetic analysis should be performed in all patients with suspected acute leukemia both at diagnosis and in follow-up. Most laboratories request that about 1 ml of aspirated bone marrow be sent in a heparinized tube for cytogenetic analysis.

- Molecular tests
  - Fluorescent *in situ* hybridization (FISH)
    - FISH analysis is more sensitive than cytogenetic analysis for the detection of specific chromosomal abnormalities.
    - In FISH analysis, a deoxyribonucleic acid (DNA) probe with an incorporated reporter molecule is hybridized to its complementary locus on a chromosome. The reporter molecule may be a protein or a fluorescent molecule.
    - FISH analysis can be used to detect numeric chromosomal abnormalities and specific translocations. Usually 200–500 cells are analyzed.
  - Polymerase chain reaction (PCR)
    - PCR techniques involve the use of oligonucleotide primers that bind to short complementary DNA sequences and serve as anchors for the synthesis of longer strands of DNA. These techniques allow for the detection of minute amounts of known DNA or RNA; a specific DNA rearrangement can be detected in one out of a million cells.

        - PCR testing is useful for monitoring patients with known translocations, including the t(15;17) that occurs in acute promyelocytic leukemia (APL).
- Lumbar puncture
    - Some centers routinely perform diagnostic lumbar punctures in all newly diagnosed patients with ALL to exclude leukemic involvement of the CNS. The value of this practice is controversial. If performed, the spinal fluid should be sent for cell count, differential, protein, glucose, and cytologic analysis of a centrifuged specimen.
    - Many treatment protocols for ALL involve the use of intrathecal chemotherapy as prophylaxis against the development of CNS leukemia. In these protocols, a lumbar puncture with injection of intrathecal chemotherapy is often performed at the beginning of induction chemotherapy.

Principles of Chemotherapy Treatment

- The first cycle of chemotherapy is called "induction" because its goal is to "induce" a complete remission (CR). CR is defined as the presence of all of the following:
    - Normalization of blood counts
    - No blasts detectable in the peripheral blood by analysis of a blood smear
    - Fewer than 5% blasts in the bone marrow
- Although CR may be achieved, relapse occurs in essentially all patients who do not receive additional chemotherapy, because undetectable leukemia cells, also known as "minimal residual disease," persist.
- To eradicate minimal residual disease, "postremission" chemotherapy is administered after induction. Postremission therapy is generally classified as "intensification," in which courses of high-dose chemotherapy are administered, or "consolidation," in which courses of chemotherapy with similar intensity to induction are administered.

- After completion of the intensification-consolidation phase, "maintenance" chemotherapy may be administered, especially in patients with ALL. Maintenance therapy consists of prolonged (1–3 years), low-dose chemotherapy designed to maintain remissions.

Preparation for Induction Chemotherapy and Supportive Care

- An echocardiogram or radionuclide ventriculography is generally performed to evaluate cardiac function before the use of anthracyclines.
- A multilumen central venous catheter is generally placed for the administration of chemotherapy, supportive medications, and transfusions.
- Growth factors
  - In a study in patients with ALL, treatment with filgrastim, also known as granulocyte colony-stimulating factor (G-CSF), led to a shorter duration of neutropenia and thrombocytopenia, fewer days in the hospital, a higher rate of CR, and fewer deaths during induction. However, disease-free survival and overall survival were not improved with the use of filgrastim. Therefore, treatment with filgrastim in patients with ALL results in minor benefits but does not ultimately improve survival.[10]
  - In patients with AML, the use of growth factors like filgrastim or sargramostim (granulocyte-macrophage colony-stimulating factor [GM-CSF]) shortens the duration of neutropenia by a few days and may reduce the rate of major infections. Multiple randomized trials, however, have not demonstrated an improvement in survival, with the exception of an Eastern Cooperative Oncology Group (ECOG) trial that used GM-CSF.[11,12]
  - Many protocols use filgrastim 5–10 μg/kg subcutaneously (SC) daily, beginning after chemotherapy has completed and continuing until the absolute neutrophil count recovers.

- Antibiotics
  - Although evidence supporting the use of prophylactic antibiotics in patients undergoing induction chemotherapy is limited, many centers use prophylactic antibacterial antibiotics (eg, quinolones), antivirals (eg, acyclovir), and antifungals (eg, fluconazole) in an attempt to minimize the risk of infection during the neutropenic period.
  - In febrile patients, cultures should be performed to identify a causative organism, and broad-spectrum antibiotics should be administered. In patients with persistent fever despite several days of broad-spectrum antibiotics, antifungal therapy such as amphotericin B, liposomal amphotericin B, or caspofungin should be considered. Antibiotics should generally be continued until the infection resolves and the neutrophil count rises above 500–1000/μL.
- Tumor lysis prophylaxis
  - Patients with acute leukemia are at risk for tumor lysis syndrome during induction chemotherapy.
  - To minimize the risk of tumor lysis syndrome, intravenous hydration and treatment with allopurinol (300–600 mg by mouth daily) are recommended. These should begin prior to chemotherapy and be continued for 1–2 weeks.
- Transfusions
  - Virtually all patients require transfusions of packed red blood cells and platelets during induction and during subsequent courses of chemotherapy.
  - Blood products should be leukocyte reduced to lower the risks of febrile nonhemolytic transfusion reactions, alloimmunization to human leukocyte antigens and the subsequent development of refractoriness to platelet transfusions, and transmission of cytomegalovirus (CMV).
  - Blood products should also be gamma irradiated to reduce the risk of transfusion-related graft-versus-host disease.
  - Platelets should generally be transfused prophylactically when the platelet count drops below 10,000/μL

or at higher thresholds when other risk factors for bleeding, such as fever, severe mucositis, or coagulopathy, are present.
- Directed donations from relatives should be avoided.

- Leukapheresis should be performed prior to or in conjunction with induction chemotherapy in patients with a markedly elevated WBC count (eg, >100,000/μL) and resulting symptoms of leukostasis.

References

1. Bennett JM, Catovsky D, Daniel MT, et al. Proposals for the classification of the acute leukaemias. French-American-British (FAB) Cooperative Group. *Br J Haematol.* 1976; 33:451-458.
2. Bennett JM, Catovsky D, Daniel MT, et al. Proposed revised criteria for the classification of acute myeloid leukemia. A report of the French-American-British Cooperative Group. *Ann Intern Med.* 1985;103:620-625.
3. Bennett JM, Catovsky D, Daniel MT, et al. Criteria for the diagnosis of acute leukemia of megakaryocyte lineage (M7). A report of the French-American-British Cooperative Group. *Ann Intern Med.* 1985;103:460-462.
4. Bennett JM, Catovsky D, Daniel MT, et al. Proposal for the recognition of minimally differentiated acute myeloid leukaemia (AML-MO). *Br J Haematol.* 1991;78:325-329.
5. Jaffe ES, Harris NL, Stein H, Vardiman JW, eds. *Pathology and Genetics of Tumours of Haematopoietic and Lymphoid Tissues*. Lyon: IARC Press; 2001.
6. Estey E, Thall P, Beran M, et al. Effect of diagnosis (refractory anemia with excess blasts, refractory anemia with excess blasts in transformation, or acute myeloid leukemia [AML]) on outcome of AML-type chemotherapy. *Blood.* 1997;90:2969-2977.
7. Greenberg P, Cox C, LeBeau MM, et al. International scoring system for evaluating prognosis in myelodysplastic syndromes. *Blood.* 1997;89:2079-2088.
8. Huh YO, Ibrahim S. Immunophenotypes in adult acute lymphocytic leukemia. Role of flow cytometry in diagnosis and monitoring of disease. *Hematol Oncol Clin North Am.* 2000;14:1251-1265.
9. Todd WM. Acute myeloid leukemia and related conditions. *Hematol Oncol Clin North Am.* 2002;16:301-319.

10. Larson RA, Dodge RK, Linker CA, et al. A randomized controlled trial of filgrastim during remission induction and consolidation chemotherapy for adults with acute lymphoblastic leukemia: CALGB study 9111. *Blood.* 1998; 92:1556-1564.
11. Rowe JM, Andersen JW, Mazza JJ, et al. A randomized placebo-controlled phase III study of granulocyte-macrophage colony-stimulating factor in adult patients (>55 to 70 years of age) with acute myelogenous leukemia: a study of the Eastern Cooperative Oncology Group (E1490). *Blood.* 1995;86:457-462.
12. Stone RM, Berg DT, George SL, et al. Granulocyte-macrophage colony-stimulating factor after initial chemotherapy for elderly patients with primary acute myelogenous leukemia. Cancer and Leukemia Group B. *N Engl J Med.* 1995;332:1671-1677.

CHAPTER 2

Acute Myeloid Leukemia

Epidemiology

- Estimated 11,960 new cases in the United States in 2005[1]
- Accounts for about 75% of cases of acute leukemia in adults
- Median age, 60 years; incidence increases after age 40 years
- M = F
- Risk factors
  - Previous chemotherapy
    - Alkylating agents
      - Associated with deletions of chromosomes 5 and 7
      - Risk for development of AML is highest between 2 and 9 years after exposure
    - Epipodophyllotoxins (eg, etoposide)
      - Associated with abnormalities of chromosome 11q23 and occasionally the t(15;17) translocation that is associated with APL
      - Risk for development of AML is highest between 1 and 3 years after exposure
  - Previous radiation exposure
  - Environmental factors (tobacco, benzene)
  - Genetic factors
    - Down's syndrome
    - Fanconi's anemia
    - Ataxia telangiectasia

Classification

- The Cooperative FAB Group proposed a widely used classification scheme that divided AML into eight different subtypes called M0–M7 (Table 2-1).[2]

Table 2-1: FAB Classification of AML

Subtype	Name	Morphology	Cytochemistry: Myeloperoxidase	Cytochemistry: Nonspecific esterase	Comments	Approximate frequency
M0	AML with minimal myeloid differentiation	≥30% of nucleated marrow cells are large, agranular myeloblasts.	–	–	Distinguished fiom ALL when immunophenotyping shows positivity for CD13 and/or CD33.	3%
M1	Myeloblastic leukemia without maturation	≥90% of nucleated marrow cells are poorly differentiated myeloblasts.	≥3%	–		20%
M2	Myeloblastic leukemia with maturation	30–89% of nucleated marrow cells are myeloblasts with granules. < 20% of cells are monocytes. Auer rods common.	+	–	Often associated with t(8;21)(q22;q22).	25%

M3	Acute promyelocytic leukemia	≥30% of nucleated marrow cells are blasts or hypergranular promyelocytes. Auer rods common.	+	–	Associated with t(15;17)(q22;q12) and other variant translocations involving *RARα* gene on chromosome 17.	10%
M4	Acute myelomonocytic leukemia	30–80% of nonerythroid cells are myeloblasts, promyelocytes, myelocytes, or other granulocytic precursor. Monocytic cells ≥ 20% of nonerythroid cells.	+/–	+	M4Eo subtype containing abnormal eosinophils with basophilic granules is associated with inv(16)(p13q22) or t(16;16)(p13;q22).	25%
M5	Acute monocytic leukemia	≥80% of nonerythroid cells are monoblasts, promonocytes, or monocytes.	–	+	Subdivided into M5a, in which ≥80% of the monocytic cells are monoblasts, and M5b, in which <80% of the	5%

Table 2-1: continued

Subtype	Name	Morphology	Cytochemistry		Comments	Approximate frequency
			Myeloperoxidase	Nonspecific esterase		
					monocytic cells are monoblasts (the rest are promonocytes and monocytes).	
M6	Acute erythroleukemia	≥50% of nucleated marrow cells are erythroid. ≥30% of nonerythroid cells are myeloblasts.	+/−	−	Erythroid precursors are frequently positive for the periodic acid-Schiff (PAS) reaction.	5%
M7	Acute megakaryoblastic leukemia	≥30% of nucleated marrow cells are megakaryoblasts.	−	−	Immunophenotyping shows positivity for CD41 orCD61.	5%

ALL, acute lymphoblastic leukemia; AML, acute myeloid leukemia; FAB, French-American-British Cooperative Group.

- More recently, the WHO proposed a revised classification scheme that incorporates important prognostic information, including cytogenetic abnormalities and whether the AML is related to prior chemotherapy exposure (Table 2-2).[3-8]

Table 2-2: World Health Organization Classification of AML

Type	Subtypes and descriptions
AML with recurrent cytogenetic abnormalities	1. AML with t(8;21)(q22;q22);(AML1/ETO) 2. AML with abnormal bone marrow eosinophils inv(16)(p13q22) or t(16;16)(p13;q22); (CBFβ/MYH11) 3. Acute promyelocytic leukemia [AML with t(15;17)(q22;q12) (PML/*RARα*) and variants] 4. AML with 11q23 (MLL) abnormalities
AML with multilineage dysplasia	1. Following a myelodysplastic syndrome or myelodysplastic syndrome/myeloproliferative disorder 2. Without antecedent myelodysplastic syndrome
AML and MDS, therapy related	1. Alkylating agent–related 2. Topoisomerase type II inhibitor–related (some may be lymphoid)
AML not otherwise categorized	1. AML minimally differentiated —Blasts do not stain with myeloperoxidase or Sudan black —Myeloid etiology demonstrated by immunophenotyping or ultrastructural studies 2. AML without maturation —Blasts $\geq$ 90% of nucleated bone marrow cells —$>$ 3% of blasts positive for MPO or SBB, or Auer rods present 3. AML with maturation —Blasts $\geq$ 20% of nucleated bone marrow cells —Evidence of maturation to more mature neutrophils ($\geq$ 10% of nucleated marrow cells are neutrophils or their precursors) —Monocytes $<$ 20% of nucleated bone marrow cells

Table 2-2: continued

Type	Subtypes and descriptions
	4. Acute myelomonocytic leukemia —Blasts ≥ 20% of nucleated bone marrow cells —≥ 20% of nucleated marrow cells are neutrophils or their precursors —≥ 20% of nucleated marrow cells are monocytes or their precursors 5. Acute monoblastic and monocytic leukemia —Blasts ≥ 20% of nucleated bone marrow cells —≥ 80% of leukemic cells are of monocytic lineage (monoblasts, promonocytes, monocytes) —Monoblastic: majority of monocytic cells are monoblasts —Monocytic: majority of monocytic cells are promonocytes 6. Acute erythroid leukemia: two subtypes —Erythroleukemia: blasts ≥ 20% of nucleated bone marrow cells and erythroid precursors ≥ 50% of nucleated bone marrow cells —Pure erythroid leukemia: blasts are not increased and erythroid precursors > 80% of marrow cells 7. Acute megakaryoblastic leukemia: ≥ 50% of blasts are of megakaryocyte lineage 8. Acute basophilic leukemia 9. Acute panmyelosis with myelofibrosis 10. Myeloid sarcoma

AML, acute myeloid leukemia; MDS, myelodysplastic syndromes; MPO, myeloperoxidase; SBB, Sudan black B; WHO, World Health Organization.

Modified with permission from Jaffe et al. *Pathology and Genetics of Tumours of Haematopoietic and Lymphoid Tissues.* Lyon: IARC Press; 2001.

- The WHO classification scheme is probably more useful to the practicing clinician, although the FAB scheme is still commonly employed.
- Occasionally, cases arise in which differentiation between AML and ALL is difficult. These are described

by the WHO as "acute leukemias of ambiguous lineage" and are divided into three subtypes:

- *Undifferentiated acute leukemia*, which lacks all of the lineage-specific markers myeloperoxidase, CD3, cytoplasmic CD22, and cytoplasmic CD79a
- *Bilineal acute leukemia*, which is characterized by a dual population of blasts, with each population expressing markers of a distinct lineage
- *Biphenotypic acute leukemia*, which is characterized by blasts that coexpress lineage-*specific* antigens from two lineages. Note that coexpression of one or two lineage-*associated* antigens from another lineage is not a sufficient criterion to diagnose biphenotypic leukemia and should instead be called either "myeloid antigen-positive ALL" or "lymphoid antigen-positive AML," depending on whether the expressed lineage-specific antigen is lymphoid or myeloid, respectively.

- As further advances are made in the development of prognostic tools, new classification schemes will undoubtedly follow.

Pathology

- Morphology
  - Myeloblasts in blood or bone marrow may vary in size from medium (ie, slightly larger than mature lymphocytes) to very large (ie, larger than a monocyte). The cytoplasm is moderate in amount (more than in lymphoblasts) and bluish in color. The chromatin is fine and granular. Nucleoli tend to be more prominent than in lymphoblasts. A few azurophilic granules may be present. Auer rods, which are reddish, spindle-shaped filaments of aggregated granules, may be present (Figure 2-1).
  - Table 2-3 lists some of the features that assist in the distinction between myeloblasts and lymphoblasts. With the exception of Auer rods, none of these features can be used to definitively distinguish myeloblasts from lymphoblasts. For this reason, cytochemistry and/or immunophenotyping is essential in all cases of acute leukemia.

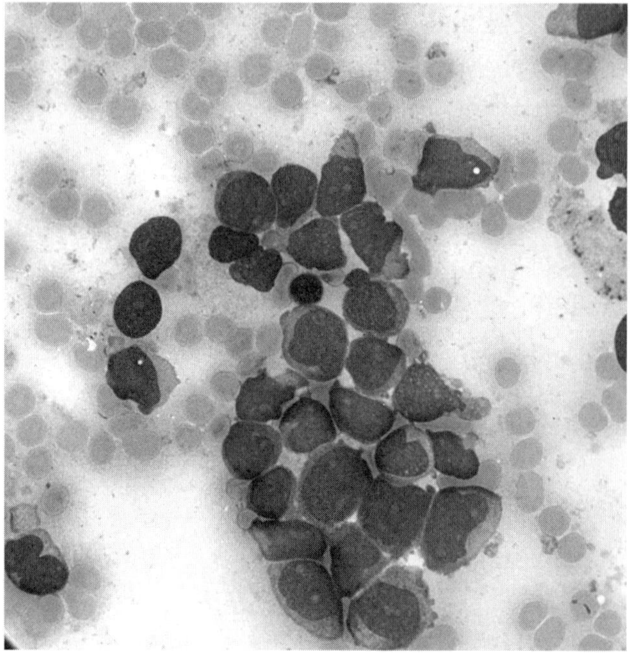

Figure 2-1: Bone marrow aspirate in a patient with acute myeloid leukemia (AML). Almost all of the nucleated cells are blasts. The blast at the top contains a small Auer rod. The myeloblasts contain more cytoplasm than is typically seen in lymphoblasts. Many of the blasts have prominent nucleoli. The patient's leukemia was classified as M1 (by the French-American-British criteria), or AML without maturation.

- Genetics
  - Principles
    - Clonal chromosomal abnormalities can be detected in about 70% of patients with AML; the other 30% of patients have a normal karyotype.[9]
    - These chromosomal abnormalities have prognostic and therapeutic significance. Therefore, cytogenetic analysis should be performed for every patient with newly diagnosed acute leukemia.

Table 2-3: Morphologic Differences Between Myeloblasts and Lymphoblasts

Characteristic	Myeloblasts	Lymphoblasts
Size	Medium-large	Small-medium
Amount of cytoplasm	Moderate	Small
Nuclear chromatin	Fine granular	Clumped
Nucleoli	Prominent	Not prominent
Auer rods	Present	Absent
Hand-mirror cells	Absent	Present

- Common abnormalities[4]
  - t(8;21)(q22;q22); (*AML1/ETO*)
    - Occurs in 5–12% of patients with AML. Patients tend to be younger.
    - Usually produces M2 subtype (AML with maturation)
    - Results in fusion of *AML1* gene, which encodes the protein core-binding factor alpha (CBFα) with the *ETO* (eight–twenty-one) gene
    - Confers a favorable prognosis when high-dose cytarabine is used in the consolidation phase of treatment
  - inv(16)(p13q22) or t(16;16)(p13;q22); (*CBFβ/MYH11*)
    - Occurs in 10–12% of patients with AML. Patients tend to be younger.
    - Usually produces M4Eo subtype (acute myelomonocytic leukemia with abnormal bone marrow eosinophils). Morphologically, promyelocytes and myelocytes contain eosinophilic granules that are abnormally large, purple-violet, and frequently quite dense (Figure 2-2).

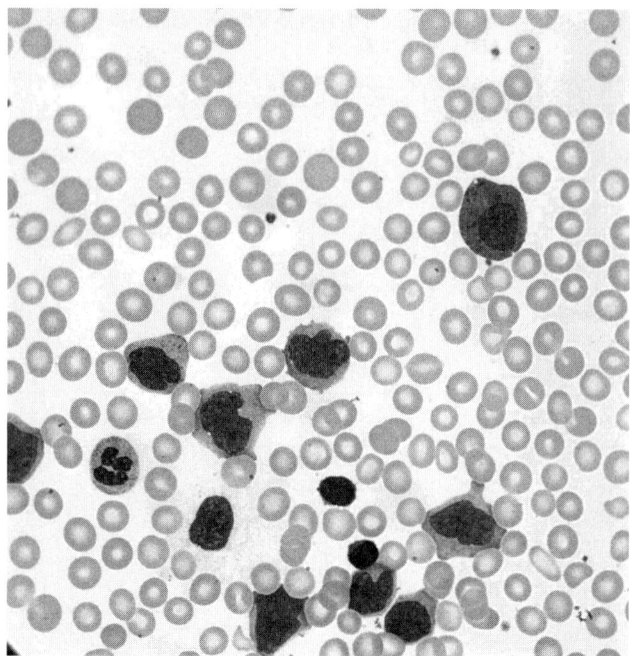

Figure 2-2: Bone marrow aspirate in a patient with acute myelomonocytic leukemia with abnormal eosinophils. The eosinophil at the top right has some large basophilic granules.

- Results in fusion of the *CBF*β gene, which encodes the β subunit of core binding factor at 16q22, to the *MYH11* gene, which encodes the smooth muscle myosin heavy chain at 16p13
- Confers a favorable prognosis when high-dose cytarabine is used in the consolidation phase of treatment

■ t(15;17)(q22;q12) (*PML/RAR*α) and variants t(11;17)(q23;q21), t(5;17)(q32;q12), and t(11;17)(q13;q21)

- Occurs in 5–8% of patients with AML
- Produces M3 subtype (APL, Figure 2-3)

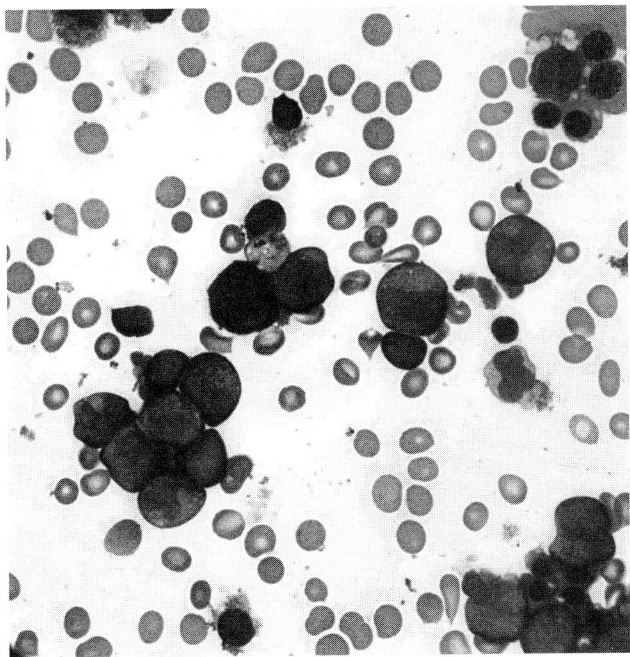

Figure 2-3: Bone marrow aspirate in a patient with acute promyelocytic leukemia. There are numerous abnormal promyelocytes containing the characteristic, heavy azurophilic granulation.

- Results in fusion of PML (promyelocytic leukemia) gene on 15q22 with
α (retinoic acid receptor alpha) gene on 17q12
- Confers a favorable prognosis. Treatment program should include all-trans retinoic acid except in patients with t(11;17)(q23;q21), in whom retinoic acid therapy is ineffective. Arsenic trioxide is also useful in this subtype

- Rearrangements involving 11q23 (*MLL*)
  - Occur in 5–6% of patients with AML. Occur frequently in infants
  - Often occur after exposure to DNA topoisomerase II inhibitors (epipodophyllotoxins)

        - Tend to produce M4 and M5 subtypes
        - Confer an intermediate prognosis
    - Others
        - Deletions of chromosome 5, deletions of chromosome 7, and trisomy 8 are commonly seen when AML evolves from a myelodysplastic syndrome.
        - Abnormalities of 3q26 are associated with increased bone marrow megakaryocytes and thrombocytosis.
- Immunophenotype[3-8]
    - Immunophenotypic analysis helps distinguish between the minimally differentiated subtype of AML (M0), in which myeloperoxidase stains are negative, and ALL.
    - It also helps identify acute megakaryoblastic leukemia (M7), because megakaryoblasts express the platelet glycoproteins CD41 (glycoprotein IIb/IIIa) and CD61 (glycoprotein IIIa).
    - Subtypes of AML may have characteristic immunophenotypic features. For example, in APL, CD33 is usually expressed, but CD34 and HLA-DR are not. This is in contrast to many other subtypes of AML, in which CD34 and HLA-DR are usually expressed together with CD33.
    - Myeloblasts tend to express CD13, CD33, HLA-DR, and CD117.
    - CD11 and CD44 may be expressed, particularly in patients with M4 (acute myelomonocytic leukemia) and M5 (acute monoblastic leukemia) subtypes.
    - Lymphoid antigens may be expressed in about 20% of cases.
    - Terminal deoxynucleotidyl transferase (TdT) is expressed in about 20% of cases.

Prognosis

- The percentage of patients achieving CR is approximately 50–70%, and the percentage of patients achieving long-term disease-free survival is approximately 20–30%.

- Three most important prognostic factors
  - Age
    - Older age is associated with lower rates of CR and long-term survival.
    - The percentage of patients older than age 60 years who achieve CR is approximately 30–50%, and the percentage alive at 5 years is less than 10%.
  - Antecedent hematologic disorder or prior exposure to chemotherapy
    - The presence of an antecedent hematologic disorder, such as myelodysplastic syndrome or a myeloproliferative disorder, lowers the rates of CR and overall survival.
    - AML that occurs as a result of prior exposure to chemotherapy has a poor prognosis.
  - Cytogenetics
    - Specific cytogenetic abnormalities correlate with favorable, intermediate, and unfavorable outcomes (Table 2-4).[10,11]
    - Recent evidence suggests that trisomy 8 as an isolated cytogenetic abnormality may be an unfavorable prognostic factor, and some centers consider this mutation as such.[12]

Table 2-4: Prognostic Value of Cytogenetic Abnormalities in Acute Myeloid Leukemia

Favorable	Intermediate	Unfavorable
t(15;17)	Normal karyotype	Complex karyotype (≥ 3 abnormalities)
t(8;21) without del(9q) or complex karyotype	+8*	del(5q), −5
inv(16), t(16;16), del(16q)	−Y	del(7q), −7
	+6	inv(3q)
	del(12p)	abn 11q23, 17p, 20q, or 21q
	All others	del(9q), t(6;9), t(9;22)

*Some evidence suggests that isolated trisomy 8 may confer an unfavorable prognosis.

Modified with permission from Appelbaum et al. *Hematology (Am Soc Hematol Educ Program).* 2001;62-86.

Treatment of AML

- Principles
  - Without treatment, AML is fatal, usually within a matter of months.
  - Chemotherapy can cure patients and prolong survival in responding patients.
  - Chemotherapy is also quite toxic and causes substantial morbidity and mortality.
  - The goal of induction chemotherapy is to "induce" a CR, defined as normalization of peripheral blood counts and bone marrow.
  - Patients in remission after induction chemotherapy have a large number of residual leukemia cells in their bodies. Without postremission therapy, essentially all patients will relapse. Some patients achieving CR are unable to receive postremission therapy because of persistent toxicity from induction therapy.
  - The goal of postremission chemotherapy is to eradicate minimal residual disease and cure the patient.
- Induction chemotherapy
  - The most commonly used induction regimen consists of cytarabine 100 mg/m^2 by intravenous continuous infusion (IVCI) daily for 7 days on days 1–7, plus either daunorubicin 45 mg/m^2 IV push daily for 3 days on days 1–3 or idarubicin 12 mg/m^2 IV push daily for 3 days on days 1–3. This is often called the "7+3" regimen.
  - In many studies, a bone marrow aspirate is performed approximately 14 days after the beginning of therapy. If greater than 5% of the nucleated cells in the marrow are blasts, a second course of induction chemotherapy identical or similar to the first (often "5+2" instead of "7+3") is given immediately. If 5% or less of the nucleated cells in the marrow are blasts, no further treatment is administered until after recovery of peripheral blood counts. Whether this approach is superior to the alternative approach of not performing a bone marrow examination at day 14 and allowing patients to recover from their initial chemotherapy has

not been demonstrated (to the author's knowledge), and at some centers the day 14 bone marrow examination is not performed.

- Whether idarubicin is superior to daunorubicin is controversial. Several randomized studies have compared the two drugs. Some have shown improved response rates and survival with idarubicin, but these differences in outcomes may have been related to inequities in dosing.[13-15]
- In two studies, disease-free survival was improved with higher doses of cytarabine; however, overall survival was not significantly affected.[16,17]
- Effects
  - 50–75% of patients younger than 60 years of age achieve CR.
  - 30–50% of patients older than 60 years of age achieve CR with standard induction, although the treatment-related mortality is about 15–20%.[18]
  - Only the minority of patients with therapy-related AML achieve CR.
  - The median duration of remission with standard induction is 8–12 months.

- Postremission chemotherapy
  - Several options exist:
    - Repeat induction, perhaps with fewer days of treatment (eg, cytarabine 100–200 mg/m^2 IVCI daily for 4 days plus idarubicin 12 mg/m^2 IV push daily for 2 days, or "4+2")
    - Low-dose cytarabine (eg, 100–200 mg/m^2 IVCI daily for 5–7 days)
    - Intermediate-dose cytarabine (eg, 1,500 mg/m^2 IV over 1 hour every 12 hours for 3–6 days)
    - High-dose cytarabine (eg, 3,000 mg/m^2 IV over 3 hours every 12 hours on days 1, 3, and 5)
  - In a Cancer and Leukemia Group B (CALGB) trial, consolidation therapy with up to four cycles of high-dose cytarabine improved 4-year disease-free survival in patients younger than 60 years of age compared with intermediate- or low-dose cytarabine. However, in patients older than 60 years of age, high-dose

cytarabine resulted in a higher toxic death rate and did not improve the disease-free survival rate (16% at 4 years) compared with lower doses of cytarabine.[19]

- Several groups have demonstrated that consolidation with high-dose cytarabine is more effective in patients with core-binding factor-type leukemias [eg, t(8;21), t(16;16), and inv(16)] than in patients with normal karyotypes or other cytogenetic abnormalities. For example, in the CALGB trial, the 5-year disease-free survival rate was 50% in patients with core-binding factor–type leukemias, 32% in patients with normal karyotypes, and 15% in patients with other cytogenetic abnormalities.[10]
- Conclusions
  - Based on these data, common practice has been to treat patients younger than 60 years of age with favorable- or intermediate-prognosis cytogenetics with up to four cycles of high-dose cytarabine as consolidation. The optimal number of cycles is unknown, and many patients will not be able to tolerate all four cycles of therapy.
  - Patients older than 60 years of age are often treated with lower doses of cytarabine, either alone or with daunorubicin or idarubicin (eg, "4+2").
  - Young patients with unfavorable-prognosis cytogenetics are often considered for transplantation-based postremission therapy.

- Autologous and allogeneic stem cell transplantation in first remission
  - Three large trials have attempted to compare conventional chemotherapy with autologous and allogeneic stem cell transplantation as postremission therapy in young patients with AML in first CR.[20-22] Neither type of transplantation improved overall survival in any of the studies.
  - Conclusions
    - Stem cell transplantation for patients with AML in first remission is not usually performed in those with favorable- or intermediate-risk cytogenetics.

    - In young patients with unfavorable-risk disease, stem cell transplantation may be considered in first remission because of the poor results with conventional chemotherapy. Whether transplantation actually improves outcomes in these patients is not clear. If a matched sibling or unrelated donor is available, allogeneic transplantation is usually performed. If not, autologous transplantation may be considered.
- Maintenance chemotherapy
  - Maintenance therapy refers to the administration of low doses of chemotherapy designed to maintain remissions without causing undue toxicity.
  - An ECOG study in the 1980s demonstrated that maintenance therapy was superior to observation in patients in CR after induction.[23]
  - A recent German study found that maintenance chemotherapy improved relapse-free but not overall survival.[24]
  - Despite these findings, maintenance chemotherapy after consolidation has not become standard practice. Nevertheless, maintenance therapy may be considered in elderly patients who cannot tolerate more intensive consolidation therapy.
- Treatment of refractory or relapsed disease
  - Principles
    - Most patients with AML relapse and die of their disease.
    - Many patients who experience relapse, especially those with long first remissions, can achieve a second CR.
    - AML that is refractory to initial induction chemotherapy or that relapses within 6 months of remission is not likely to be cured with conventional chemotherapy. The preferred treatment for these patients is high-dose chemotherapy followed by allogeneic transplantation.
    - Treatment options

        - Conventional chemotherapy drugs: anthracyclines, cytarabine, etoposide, fludarabine, topotecan, and others may be used
        - Gemtuzumab ozogamicin (see below)
        - High-dose therapy with allogeneic transplantation: the preferred treatment approach in young patients with relapsed AML and available HLA-matched donors
- Gemtuzumab ozogamicin (GO) (Mylotarg®)
    - Mechanism
        - GO is a recombinant humanized anti-CD33 antibody conjugated to calicheamicin, a cytotoxic antitumor antibiotic.
        - After administration, GO is internalized into lysosomes, where the calicheamicin dissociates from the antibody. Calicheamicin then migrates to the nucleus and causes double-stranded DNA breaks.
    - Efficacy[25]
        - In a study of patients with AML in first relapse whose remissions lasted at least 3 months, treatment with GO resulted in CR in 16% of patients and in CR except for incomplete platelet recovery in an additional 13% of patients.
        - Median survival was 5.9 months, and the overall survival rate at 1 year was 31%.
    - Toxicities: fever, chills, dyspnea, hypotension, nausea/vomiting, mucositis, myelosuppression, hyperbilirubinemia and elevated transaminases, veno-occlusive disease of the liver, acute respiratory distress syndrome
    - Dose: 9 mg/m^2 IV over 2 hours on days 1 and 15. Leukoreduction with leukapheresis or hydroxyurea is recommended to lower the WBC count below 30,000/μL prior to therapy. Acetaminophen and diphenhydramine should be administered as premedications. Measures to prevent tumor lysis syndrome are recommended.
    - FDA approval: based on these data, the FDA approved GO for the treatment of patients aged 60

years or older with CD33-positive AML in first relapse who are not considered candidates for cytotoxic chemotherapy.
- Future directions: current studies are investigating GO in conjunction with other chemotherapy drugs and in other settings such as during induction and as maintenance therapy.

- Treatment of elderly patients
  - Not all patients should receive chemotherapy for AML. Elderly patients with significant comorbidities and poor performance status sometimes should receive only supportive care. In this way, treatment must be individualized.
  - Outcomes in elderly patients with AML are worse than in younger patients with AML. In otherwise healthy patients older than 60 years of age, the rate of CR with standard induction is 30–50%, and the 5-year survival rate is about 10%. Treatment-related mortality is about 15–20%.[18]
  - High-dose cytarabine is more toxic in patients older than 60 years of age and generally should not be used as postremission therapy.
  - Options for postremission therapy in otherwise healthy elderly patients include a "4+2" regimen or intermediate doses of cytarabine (eg, 1,500 mg/m^2 intravenous piggyback [IVPB] over 3 hours q 12 hours × 6 doses).
  - The optimal number of postremission chemotherapy cycles to administer is unknown; two are often administered, assuming the patient tolerates them well.
  - G-CSF or GM-CSF is usually used to support elderly patients during chemotherapy cycles.

Treatment of APL

- Principles
  - APL is a unique subtype of AML for a number of reasons:
    - Characteristic cytogenetic abnormalities—t(15;17) and variants—are present. The PML-RARα transcript that results from this translocation can be

detected in peripheral blood and bone marrow by polymerase chain reaction (PCR) testing.
  - The rate of disseminated intravascular coagulopathy and bleeding complications is high compared with other subtypes of AML. Transfusion of platelets for thrombocytopenia and of cryoprecipitate for hypofibrinogenemia is necessary for many patients.
  - All-trans retinoic acid and arsenic trioxide are particularly effective drugs. When administered in combination with chemotherapy, retinoic acid results in higher rates of remission and disease-free survival than are seen in other subtypes of AML.
- Prognosis
  - Adverse prognostic factors at presentation[26]
    - High WBC count (cutoff ranges from 2,000–10,000/μL)
    - Low platelet count (< 40,000/μL)
    - Male sex
    - CD56 expression
  - After induction, approximately 50–60% of patients are PCR-negative. More than 90% of patients are PCR-negative after two cycles of consolidation.[27,28]
  - With modern regimens, approximately 50–75% of patients achieve long-term disease-free survival.
- All-trans retinoic acid
  - Mechanism: causes maturation of the abnormal cell clone, leading to differentiation and eventually apopototic cell death.
  - Efficacy
    - As a single agent, retinoic acid results in high rates of CR, although the durations of remission are usually short (ie, months).
    - Patients with morphological features of APL but who are PML/RARα-negative generally have disease refractory to retinoic acid.
    - Differs from chemotherapy in the following ways:

  - Does not cause bone marrow aplasia
  - Improves coagulation parameters within a few days, whereas chemotherapy may worsen them
  - May cause leukocytosis, which in turn may be associated with the retinoic acid syndrome
  - Unique side effect is "retinoic acid syndrome"
- Retinoic acid syndrome
  - Incidence: rate is about 25% when retinoic acid is used alone, but only 10% when retinoic acid is used together with chemotherapy
  - Clinical features: fever, dyspnea, peripheral edema with weight gain, pleural effusions, pericardial effusions, hypotension, renal failure. If untreated, it can lead to rapid clinical deterioration and death.
  - Treatment: stop retinoic acid and start dexamethasone 10 mg IV two or three times daily for 3 or more days.

- Induction
  - Two randomized studies have demonstrated that the addition of retinoic acid to chemotherapy during induction improves outcomes, including event-free and overall survival, compared with the use of chemotherapy alone.[29,30]
  - In the European APL93 study, concurrent retinoic acid plus chemotherapy, as compared with sequential retinoic acid followed by chemotherapy, resulted in a decreased rate of relapse and a trend toward improved event-free survival at 2 years. However, there was no difference in overall survival.[31]
  - Evidence is beginning to accumulate that the addition of cytarabine to an anthracycline plus retinoic acid in induction may not be necessary,[28,32] although this observation has not been confirmed in a randomized trial.

- Outside the setting of a clinical trial, a reasonable induction regimen to use is the Italian "AIDA" regimen (retinoic acid 22.5 mg/m^2 [12.5 mg/m^2 if aged < 20 years] by mouth twice daily until complete hematologic remission or for a maximum of 90 days, plus idarubicin 12 mg/m^2 IV daily on days 2, 4, 6, and 8).[27] In the modified regimen used by the Spanish PETHEMA group, the idarubicin dose on day 8 was omitted in patients older than 70 years of age.[28]

- Consolidation
  - Because detection of the PML-RARα transcript by PCR predicts relapse, the goal of induction and consolidation therapy is to eliminate minimal residual disease as detected by PCR analysis.
  - Although the ideal number of courses of consolidation chemotherapy alone is unknown, at least two courses are given in most protocols.
  - Most protocols have incorporated cytarabine in consolidation, although the PETHEMA group did not and still achieved excellent outcomes (approximately 80% 3-year survival rate).[28]
  - Reasonable consolidation regimens to use outside the setting of a clinical trial include the Italian AIDA regimen,[27] the North American Intergroup regimen,[30] the European APL93 regimen,[31] and the Spanish PETHEMA regimen,[28] among others.
- Maintenance
  - Two studies have suggested a role for maintenance therapy in APL.
    - In the North American Intergroup study, patients treated with 1 year of maintenance retinoic acid therapy had improved 3-year disease-free survival rates compared with patients under observation alone (65% vs. 40%, respectively).[30]
    - In the European APL93 study, patients treated with maintenance therapy had improved overall survival. Of the maintenance options, 2 years of retinoic acid plus chemotherapy with oral 6-mercaptopurine and methotrexate resulted in the lowest relapse rate.[31]

- A recent North American Intergroup study compared retinoic acid alone with retinoic acid plus chemotherapy as maintenance therapy. Results of the study are not yet available.
- Outside of a clinical trial, maintenance therapy with 1 year of retinoic acid 22.5 mg/m^2 by mouth twice daily, 2 years of retinoic acid 22.5 mg/m^2 by mouth twice daily for 15 days every 3 months, or 2 years of the latter retinoic acid regimen plus 6-mercapto-purine 90 mg/m^2 by mouth daily and methotrexate 15 mg/m^2 by mouth weekly is reasonable.

- Relapsed APL
  - A PCR test that converts from negative to persistently positive predicts clinical relapse. If this PCR conversion occurs, treatment for relapsed disease is generally initiated immediately, rather than waiting for clinical relapse.
  - Options outside the setting of a clinical trial
    - Reinduction using retinoic acid alone or with chemotherapy, particularly if the duration from last exposure to retinoic acid is greater than 6 months
    - Arsenic trioxide
  - Arsenic trioxide
    - In general, arsenic trioxide is the treatment of choice for patients with relapsed APL, especially those whose disease is resistant to retinoic acid.
    - Mechanism: induces differentiation and apoptosis of the leukemic promyelocyte
    - Efficacy: in patients with relapsed APL, the rate of CR is 85%, and the rate of PCR negativity after two courses is 78%.[33]
    - Dose
      - Induction
        - 0.15 mg/kg IV over 2 hours daily until bone marrow remission occurs, up to a cumulative maximum of 60 doses.
        - Bone marrow aspirates should be obtained on or before day 28 of therapy, then weekly until bone marrow CR.

        - Consolidation
            - Begins 3 to 4 weeks after completion of induction therapy
            - 0.15 mg/kg IV over 2 hours daily or on weekdays only, for a cumulative total of 25 doses
    - Side effects include:
        - Prolongation of the QTc interval (may cause sudden death). Monitoring with electrocardiograms performed at least weekly is recommended.
        - APL differentiation syndrome (a cardiorespiratory distress syndrome with pulmonary infiltrates, reminiscent of the retinoic acid syndrome, and responsive to dexamethasone).
  - Stem cell transplantation
    - Many patients who achieve a second CR after therapy with arsenic trioxide eventually experience relapse.
    - Patients in a second molecular remission may achieve long-term disease-free survival with autologous stem cell transplantation.[34]
    - In patients who experience relapse and achieve a second CR, high-dose therapy with autologous or allogeneic stem cell transplantation should be considered, although the evidence supporting the use of these modalities is limited.
- Follow-up[26]
  - A persistently positive reverse transcriptase (RT)-PCR test after consolidation predicts subsequent hematologic relapse, whereas a persistently negative RT-PCR test predicts long-term survival in most patients.
  - A reasonable schedule of testing is to obtain a bone marrow sample at the end of treatment; then every 3 months for the first 2 years of remission; then every 6 months for the next 2 to 3 years.

References

1. Jemal A, Murray T, Ward E, et al. Cancer statistics, 2005. *CA Cancer J Clin.* 2005;55:10-30.

2. Bennett JM, Catovsky D, Daniel MT, et al. Proposed revised criteria for the classification of acute myeloid leukemia. A report of the French-American-British Cooperative Group. *Ann Intern Med.* 1985;103:620-625.
3. Brunning RD, Matutes E, Harris NL, et al. Acute myeloid leukaemia: introduction. In: Jaffe ES, Harris NL, Stein H, Vardiman JW, eds. *Pathology and Genetics of Tumours of Haematopoietic and Lymphoid Tissues.* Lyon: IARC Press; 2001:77-80.
4. Brunning RD, Matutes E, Flandrin G, et al. Acute myeloid leukaemia with recurrent genetic abnormalities. In: Jaffe ES, Harris NL, Stein H, Vardiman JW, eds. *Pathology and Genetics of Tumours of Haematopoietic and Lymphoid Tissues.* Lyon: IARC Press; 2001:81-87.
5. Brunning RD, Matutes E, Harris NL, et al. Acute myeloid leukaemia with multilineage dysplasia. In: Jaffe ES, Harris NL, Stein H, Vardiman JW, eds. *Pathology and Genetics of Tumours of Haematopoietic and Lymphoid Tissues.* Lyon: IARC Press; 2001:88-89.
6. Brunning RD, Matutes E, Flandrin G, et al. Acute myeloid leukaemias and myelodysplastic syndromes, therapy related. In: Jaffe ES, Harris NL, Stein H, Vardiman JW, eds. *Pathology and Genetics of Tumours of Haematopoietic and Lymphoid Tissues.* Lyon: IARC Press; 2001:89-91.
7. Brunning RD, Matutes E, Flandrin G, et al. Acute myeloid leukaemia not otherwise categorised. In: Jaffe ES, Harris NL, Stein H, Vardiman JW, eds. *Pathology and Genetics of Tumours of Haematopoietic and Lymphoid Tissues.* Lyon: IARC Press; 2001:91-105.
8. Brunning RD, Matutes E, Borowitz M, et al. Acute leukaemias of ambiguous lineage. In: Jaffe ES, Harris NL, Stein H, Vardiman JW, eds. *Pathology and Genetics of Tumours of Haematopoietic and Lymphoid Tissues.* Lyon: IARC Press; 2001:106-107.
9. Tallman MS, Nabhan C. Acute myeloid leukemia and myelodysplasia. In: George JN, Williams ME, eds. *ASH-SAP American Society of Hematology Self-Assessment Program*. Malden, MA: Blackwell Publishing; 2003:165-189.
10. Bloomfield CD, Lawrence D, Byrd JC, et al. Frequency of prolonged remission duration after high-dose cytarabine intensification in acute myeloid leukemia varies by cytogenetic subtype. *Cancer Res.* 1998;58:4173-4179.

11. Grimwade D, Walker H, Oliver F, et al. The importance of diagnostic cytogenetics on outcome in AML: analysis of 1,612 patients entered into the MRC AML 10 trial. The Medical Research Council Adult and Children's Leukaemia Working Parties. *Blood.* 1998;92:2322-2333.
12. Byrd JC, Mrozek K, Dodge RK, et al. Pretreatment cytogenetic abnormalities are predictive of induction success, cumulative incidence of relapse, and overall survival in adult patients with de novo acute myeloid leukemia: results from Cancer and Leukemia Group B (CALGB 8461). *Blood.* 2002;100:4325-4336.
13. Berman E, Heller G, Santorsa J, et al. Results of a randomized trial comparing idarubicin and cytosine arabinoside with daunorubicin and cytosine arabinoside in adult patients with newly diagnosed acute myelogenous leukemia. *Blood.* 1991;77:1666-1674.
14. Vogler WR, Velez-Garcia E, Weiner RS, et al. A phase III trial comparing idarubicin and daunorubicin in combination with cytarabine in acute myelogenous leukemia: a Southeastern Cancer Study Group study. *J Clin Oncol.* 1992;10:1103-1111.
15. Wiernik PH, Banks PL, Case DC Jr, et al. Cytarabine plus idarubicin or daunorubicin as induction and consolidation therapy for previously untreated adult patients with acute myeloid leukemia. *Blood.* 1992;79:313-319.
16. Bishop JF, Matthews JP, Young GA, et al. A randomized study of high-dose cytarabine in induction in acute myeloid leukemia. *Blood.* 1996;87:1710-1717.
17. Weick JK, Kopecky KJ, Appelbaum FR, et al. A randomized investigation of high-dose versus standard-dose cytosine arabinoside with daunorubicin in patients with previously untreated acute myeloid leukemia: a Southwest Oncology Group study. *Blood.* 1996;88:2841-2851.
18. Rowe JM, Neuberg D, Friedenberg W, et al. A phase 3 study of three induction regimens and of priming with GM-CSF in older adults with acute myeloid leukemia: a trial by the Eastern Cooperative Oncology Group. *Blood.* 2004;103:479-485.
19. Mayer RJ, Davis RB, Schiffer CA, et al. Intensive postremission chemotherapy in adults with acute myeloid leukemia. Cancer and Leukemia Group B. *N Engl J Med.* 1994;331:896-903.
20. Zittoun RA, Mandelli F, Willemze R, et al. Autologous or allogeneic bone marrow transplantation compared with

intensive chemotherapy in acute myelogenous leukemia. European Organization for Research and Treatment of Cancer (EORTC) and the Gruppo Italiano Malattie Ematologiche Maligne dell'Adulto (GIMEMA) Leukemia Cooperative Groups. *N Engl J Med.* 1995;332:217-223.

21. Harousseau JL, Cahn JY, Pignon B, et al. Comparison of autologous bone marrow transplantation and intensive chemotherapy as postremission therapy in adult acute myeloid leukemia. The Groupe Ouest Est Leucemies Aigues Myeloblastiques (GOELAM). *Blood.* 1997;90:2978-2986.
22. Cassileth PA, Harrington DP, Appelbaum FR, et al. Chemotherapy compared with autologous or allogeneic bone marrow transplantation in the management of acute myeloid leukemia in first remission. *N Engl J Med.* 1998;339:1649-1656.
23. Cassileth PA, Harrington DP, Hines JD, et al. Maintenance chemotherapy prolongs remission duration in adult acute nonlymphocytic leukemia. *J Clin Oncol.* 1988;6:583-587.
24. Buchner T, Hiddemann W, Berdel WE, et al. 6-Thioguanine, cytarabine, and daunorubicin (TAD) and high-dose cytarabine and mitoxantrone (HAM) for induction, TAD for consolidation, and either prolonged maintenance by reduced monthly TAD or TAD-HAM-TAD and one course of intensive consolidation by sequential HAM in adult patients at all ages with de novo acute myeloid leukemia (AML): a randomized trial of the German AML Cooperative Group. *J Clin Oncol.* 2003;21:4496-4504.
25. Sievers EL, Larson RA, Stadtmauer EA, et al. Efficacy and safety of gemtuzumab ozogamicin in patients with CD33-positive acute myeloid leukemia in first relapse. *J Clin Oncol.* 2001;19:3244-3254.
26. Tallman MS, Nabhan C, Feusner JH, Rowe JM. Acute promyelocytic leukemia: evolving therapeutic strategies. *Blood.* 2002;99:759-767.
27. Mandelli F, Diverio D, Avvisati G, et al. Molecular remission in PML/RAR alpha-positive acute promyelocytic leukemia by combined all-trans retinoic acid and idarubicin (AIDA) therapy. Gruppo Italiano-Malattie Ematologiche Maligne dell'Adulto and Associazione Italiana di Ematologia ed Oncologia Pediatrica Cooperative Groups. *Blood.* 1997; 90:1014-1021.
28. Sanz MA, Martin G, Gonzalez M, et al. Risk-adapted treatment of acute promyelocytic leukemia with all-

trans-retinoic acid and anthracycline monochemotherapy: a multicenter study by the PETHEMA group. *Blood.* 2004; 103:1237-1243.

29. Fenaux P, Le Deley MC, Castaigne S, et al. Effect of all transretinoic acid in newly diagnosed acute promyelocytic leukemia. Results of a multicenter randomized trial. European APL 91 Group. *Blood.* 1993;82:3241-3249.
30. Tallman MS, Andersen JW, Schiffer CA, et al. All-trans-retinoic acid in acute promyelocytic leukemia. *N Engl J Med.* 1997;337:1021-1028.
31. Fenaux P, Chastang C, Chevret S, et al. A randomized comparison of all transretinoic acid (ATRA) followed by chemotherapy and ATRA plus chemotherapy and the role of maintenance therapy in newly diagnosed acute promyelocytic leukemia. The European APL Group. *Blood.* 1999;94:1192-1200.
32. Estey E, Thall PF, Pierce S, Kantarjian H, Keating M. Treatment of newly diagnosed acute promyelocytic leukemia without cytarabine. *J Clin Oncol.* 1997;15:483-490.
33. Soignet SL, Frankel SR, Douer D, et al. United States multicenter study of arsenic trioxide in relapsed acute promyelocytic leukemia. *J Clin Oncol.* 2001;19:3852-3860.
34. Lo Coco F, Diverio D, Avvisati G, et al. Therapy of molecular relapse in acute promyelocytic leukemia. *Blood.* 1999;94:2225-2229.

CHAPTER 3

Myelodysplastic Syndromes

Definition[1]

- The myelodysplastic syndromes (MDSs) are a group of acquired clonal hematopoietic stem cell diseases with the following characteristics:
    - A normocellular or hypercellular bone marrow, with cells displaying overt morphological abnormalities (ie, dysplasia)
    - Pancytopenia and a low reticulocyte count
    - Ineffective hematopoiesis in one or more of the myeloid cell lines (erythrocytic, granulocytic, or megakaryocytic)
- These syndromes may progress to AML.

Epidemiology

- Incidence: 3 cases/100,000 persons per year, but rises to 20 cases/100,000 persons over the age of 70 years per year
- Median age at diagnosis is 70 years
- M:F = 1.5:1
- Risk factors: most patients diagnosed with MDS will not have any of these known risk factors:
    - Genetic disorders
        - Down's syndrome
        - Fanconi's anemia
    - Chemicals and drugs: alkylating agents, benzene exposure
    - Radiation exposure
    - Aplastic anemia: about 50% of patients with aplastic anemia treated with immunosuppressive agents develop MDS years later

Classification

- The FAB classification scheme of 1982 divided MDS into five subtypes (Table 3-1).[2]

Table 3-1: FAB Classification of Myelodysplastic Syndromes

FAB type	% Blasts in blood	% Blasts in marrow	% Ringed sideroblasts	Blood monocytes
Refractory anemia	<1	<5	<15	rare
Refractory anemia with ringed sideroblasts	<1	<5	>15	rare
Refractory anemia with excess blasts	<5	5–20	<15	rare
Refractory anemia with excess blasts in transformation	>5	21–30	<15	variable
Chronic myelomonocytic leukemia	<5	1–20	<15	$>10^9/L$

FAB, French-American-British Cooperative Group.

Modified with permission from Fauci et al. *Harrison's Principles of Internal Medicine.* 14th ed. New York, NY: McGraw-Hill; 1998:672-679.

- More recently, the WHO classification scheme has divided MDS into eight subtypes (Table 3-2).[3] In addition, the WHO classification scheme has added a group of diseases that have overlapping features of MDS and myeloproliferative disorders; these are called "myelodysplastic/myeloproliferative diseases." The myelodysplastic/myeloproliferative diseases, particularly chronic myelomonocytic leukemia, are discussed in Chapter 6.

Pathogenesis[4]

- MDS results from neoplastic transformation of the hematopoietic stem cell, with resulting abnormal development of the myeloid lineages.
- The abnormal myeloid cells proliferate and differentiate but do not mature normally. This abnormal maturation is referred to as *ineffective hematopoiesis*.
- Myeloid precursor cells also undergo an increased rate of apoptosis in the bone marrow.
- The ineffective hematopoiesis and increased rate of apoptosis result in the production of an inadequate number of mature blood cells.

Pathology

- Morphology[3,4]
    - Peripheral blood: in patients presenting with cytopenias of unclear cause, examination of the peripheral blood smear may give clues as to the presence of MDS. Even in the presence of these abnormalities, examination of the bone marrow is still required to make a definitive diagnosis of a subtype of MDS.
        - Erythrocytes
            - Usually normocytic or macrocytic (mean corpuscular volume often elevated)
            - Anisocytosis and poikilocytosis may be present.
        - Neutrophils (Figure 3-1)
            - Hypolobulated nuclei (ie, one or two lobes instead of the usual four) may be present. These neutrophils are called pseudo-Pelger-Huet cells.

Table 3-2: World Health Organization Classification of Myelodysplastic Syndromes

WHO type	Blood findings	Marrow findings
Refractory anemia (RA)	Anemia No or rare blasts No Auer rods	Only erythroid dysplasia <5% blasts <15% ringed sideroblasts No Auer rods
Refractory anemia with ringed sideroblasts	Anemia No blasts No Auer rods	Same as RA except ≥15% ringed sideroblasts
Refractory cytopenia with multilineage dysplasia (RCMD)	2–3 cytopenias No or rare blasts No Auer rods <1,000 monocytes/μL	Same as RA except dysplasia in ≥10% of cells in ≥2 lines
Refractory cytopenia with multilineage dysplasia and ringed sideroblasts	Same as RCMD	Same as RCMD except ≥15% ringed sideroblasts
Refractory anemia with excess blasts-1	Cytopenias <5% blasts No Auer rods <1,000 monocytes/μL	Uni- or multilineage dysplasia 5–9% blasts No Auer rods

Refractory anemia with excess blasts-2	Cytopenias 5–19% blasts Auer rods	Uni- or multilineage dysplasia 10–19% blasts ± Auer rods
Unclassified MDS	Same as RCMD	Unilineage dysplasia <5% blasts No Auer rods
MDS associated with isolated del(5q)	Anemia Platelets normal or increased <5% blasts	Normal to increased dysplastic megakaryocytes <5% blasts No Auer rods

MDS, myelodysplastic syndrome; WHO, World Health Organization.

Modified with permission from Jaffe et al. *Pathology and Genetics of Tumors of Haematopoietic and Lymphoid Tissues.* Lyon: IARC Press; 2001.

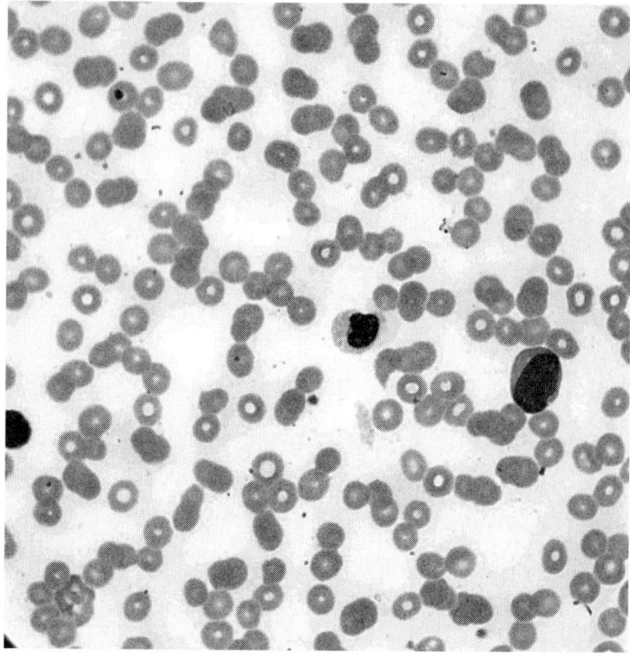

Figure 3-1: Peripheral blood smear of a patient with myelodysplastic syndrome. The neutrophil in the center is dysplastic in that the number of cytoplasmic granules is decreased and the nucleus contains only one lobe. The cell on the right is a blast. Platelets are decreased in number.

        - A decrease in the amount and number of intracytoplasmic granules, also known as "hypogranular neutrophils," may be noted.
        - Immature granulocytes (ie, "left shift") may occur. In the subtypes of MDS with excess blasts, blasts may be noted in the peripheral blood.
    - Platelets: may be large and agranular
- Bone marrow
    - Cellularity
        - The cellularity of the bone marrow in MDS is usually normal or increased.
        - Rarely, the bone marrow may be hypocellular. Historically, this has been called the "hypocel-

lular variant" of MDS. In the WHO classification, the "hypocellular variant" would fall into the "myelodysplastic syndrome, unclassifiable" category.

- Dysplastic changes: may involve one (unilineage dysplasia) or more than one (multilineage dysplasia) cell line. Unilineage dysplasia most commonly involves the erythroid series but may also occur in granulocytes and megakaryocytes. Dysplastic changes that may be observed are listed below.
    - Erythroid series
        - Nuclear abnormalities
            - Multinucleation
            - Nuclear fragmentation
            - Bizarre nuclear shape
            - Abnormal mitosis
            - Internuclear bridging
            - Abnormally dense chromatin
        - Cytoplasmic abnormalities
            - Howell-Jolly bodies
            - Defective hemoglobinization
            - Ringed sideroblasts
            - Nuclear-cytoplasmic asynchrony: dense chromatin nucleus with poorly hemoglobinized cytoplasm (megaloblastic changes)
    - Granulocytic series
        - Hypolobulation (pseudo-Pelger-Huet cells)
        - Hypogranulation
    - Megakaryocytes
        - Small megakaryocytes
        - Megakaryocytes with multiple small, widely separated nuclei
        - Hypolobulation

- Genetics
    - Approximately 50% of patients with primary MDS and 75% of patients with therapy-related MDS have chromosomal abnormalities.
    - Many of these chromosomal abnormalities have prognostic significance.

Table 3-3: Common Cytogenetic Abnormalities in Myelodysplasia

Abnormality	Incidence (%)
Loss of all or part of chromosome 5	13
Loss of all or part of chromosome 7	5
Trisomy 8	5
del(17p)	<1
del(20q)	2
Loss of X or Y	2

Reprinted with permission from Heaney and Golde. Myelodysplasia. *N Engl J Med.* 1999;340:1649-1660.

- Table 3-3 lists common chromosomal abnormalities in MDS and their frequency.

Clinical Features

- Symptoms
  - Many patients are asymptomatic and are found to have leukopenia, anemia, thrombocytopenia, or any combination of cytopenias on complete blood counts done for other reasons.
  - Symptoms from these cytopenias (eg, infections from neutropenia, fatigue from anemia, bleeding from thrombocytopenia) may be the presenting feature.
- Signs: hepatomegaly, splenomegaly, and lymphadenopathy are rare
- 5q− syndrome: MDS with isolated del(5q) has characteristic clinical features
  - Occurs more commonly in middle-aged or older women
  - Anemia is macrocytic.
  - Platelets are normal or increased in number.

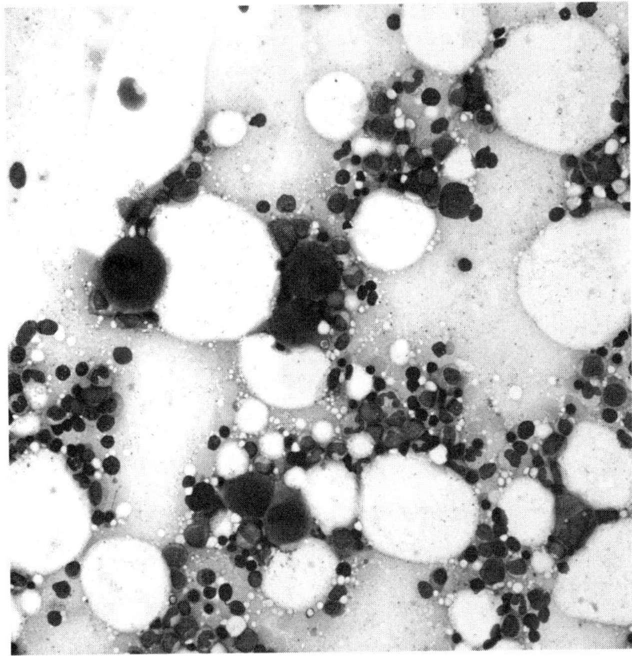

Figure 3-2: Bone marrow aspirate from a patient with 5q− syndrome. Megakaryocytes are abundant but have hypolobated nuclei.

- Megakaryocytes are abundant but dysplastic, with hypolobulated nuclei (Figure 3-2).
- Median survival is relatively long.

Course and Prognosis

- The natural history of MDS varies by the subtype (Table 3-4).
  - Patients with refractory anemia (RA) and refractory anemia with ringed sideroblasts (RARS) have a relatively low rate of progression to acute leukemia and long median survival. Progressive worsening of anemia and bone marrow failure may occur over time.
  - Patients with refractory anemia with excess blasts (RAEB-1 and RAEB-2) have a relatively high rate of

Table 3-4: Median Survival and Rate of Progression to Acute Leukemia by Subtype of MDS

MDS subtype	Rate of progression to acute leukemia (%)	Median survival (mo)
RA	6	66
RARS	1–2	72
RCMD	11	33
RAEB-1	25	18
RAEB-2	33	10
5q- syndrome	25	Favorable

MDS, myelodysplastic syndrome.

Data are from Jaffe ES, et al. *Pathology and Genetics of Tumours of Haematopoietic and Lymphoid Tissues.* Lyon: IARC Press; 2001; and from Heaney and Golde. Myelodysplasia. *N Engl J Med.* 1999;340:1649-1660.

progression to AML (≥20% blasts in the bone marrow) and short median survival. Bone marrow failure is common.

- Patients with MDS associated with del(5q) ("5q− syndrome") have a favorable prognosis with a median survival measured in years.

- Prognostic factors
  - Adverse
    - Older age
    - Increasing percentage of blasts in bone marrow
    - Increasing number of cytopenias
    - Certain cytogenetic abnormalities: abnormalities of chromosome 7 and complex (≥3) abnormalities
  - Favorable
    - Normal karyotype, del(5q), del(20q), and −Y
- International Prognostic Scoring System (IPSS) for MDS
  - The International Myelodysplastic Syndrome Working Group developed a scoring system, based on the prog-

nostic factors listed above, for predicting survival and the risk of evolution to acute leukemia (Table 3-5).[5]

- In the IPSS, patients are classified as low risk, intermediate-1 risk, intermediate-2 risk, or high risk.
- Risk stratification of patients using the IPSS can help the physician and patient make decisions about treatment.

Table 3-5: International Prognostic Scoring System for Meylodysplastic Syndromes*

Prognostic factor	Points
Percentage of blasts	
<5%	0
5–10%	0.5
11–20%	1.5
21–30%	2
Cytogenetic features	
Normal karyotype, -Y, 5q-, 20q-	0
Other	0.5
Abnormal chromosome 7, ≥ 3 abnormalities	1
Cytopenia*	
0–1 type	0
2–3 types	0.5

*Cytopenias: hemoglobin < 10 g/dL, neutrophils < 1,500/μL, platelets < 100,000/μL.

Overall score	Name	Median survival, age <70 (y)	Median survival, age >70 (y)
0	Low	9.0	3.9
0.5–1	Intermediate-1	4.4	2.4
1.5–2	Intermediate-2	1.3	1.2
≥2.5	High	0.4	0.4

Data are from Greenberg et al. *Blood.* 1997;89:2079-2088.

- One limitation of the IPSS is that patients with 21–30% blasts are described as having MDS, whereas in the new WHO classification scheme, these patients have AML.

Differential Diagnosis

- Deficiencies of vitamin B_6, B_{12}, and folate (cause megaloblastic anemia)
- Aplastic anemia
- Paroxysmal nocturnal hemoglobinuria
- Hypersplenism

Diagnostic Evaluation

- Levels of vitamin B_{12} and folate should be measured to exclude deficiency.
- CBC with differential and examination of peripheral blood smear
- Bone marrow aspirate and biopsy, conventional karyotyping, and FISH analysis for common mutations that may not be detected by conventional karyotyping

Treatment

- Observation: a reasonable approach in patients with low-risk disease who do not require transfusions
- Transfusions
    - Many patients with MDS require transfusions of erythrocytes and platelets to maintain an adequate quality of life and to avoid complications of severe anemia and thrombocytopenia.
        - Chronic transfusions may result in iron overload. When iron overload occurs, iron chelation with deferoxamine may be necessary.
- Growth factors
    - Erythropoietin
        - Efficacy
            - Increases hemoglobin levels in about 15–25% of patients

   - Decreases transfusion requirements in about 5–10% of patients
   - The response rate is related to the serum erythropoietin level; patients with serum erythropoietin levels greater than 500 mU/mL are less likely to benefit.
  - Formulations: both epoeitin alfa (Procrit®) and darbepoietin alfa (Aranesp®) are available for use, although the former has been studied more extensively.
  - Epoeitin alfa dosing options
    - 150–300 U/kg SC daily
    - 20,000 U SC three times weekly
    - 40,000 U SC weekly, but the effect of this schedule is not known
- Filgrastim (G-CSF) and sargramostim (GM-CSF)
  - Efficacy
    - Improve neutrophil counts in 80–90% of neutropenic patients and may thereby reduce the risk of infectious complications
    - In conjunction with epoeitin alfa, filgrastim improves the erythroid response rate to approximately 40%.[6]
  - Dosing of filgrastim: doses are usually adjusted to maintain a normal WBC count. Doses of 75–100 μg/day may be sufficient.
  - Indications (debatable)
    - Anemia not responding to epoeitin alfa
    - Neutropenic patients with infections
    - Absolute neutrophil count less than 200/μL

- Vitamin therapy: ineffective hematopoiesis may deplete the body's stores of vitamin B_6, B_{12}, and folate. Therefore, these are commonly administered, although responses to these are rare.
- Azacytidine (Vidaza®)
  - Mechanism
    - The enzyme DNA methyltransferase adds a methyl group to cytosine residues of newly synthesized DNA. This process decreases gene transcription.

    - Azacytidine replaces cytosine residues in newly synthesized DNA and blocks DNA methyltransferase, thereby causing "hypomethylation" of the DNA and increased gene transcription.
  - Efficacy
    - Compared with supportive care, azacytidine improves response rates, decreases transfusion requirements, improves quality of life, and decreases the rate of progression to AML. However, overall survival is not affected.[7,8]
    - Based on these data, the FDA approved azacytidine for the treatment of MDS in June 2004.
  - Dose: 75 mg/m^2 SC daily for 7 days. Repeat cycle every 28 days for up to four cycles. Doses may need to be adjusted in patients with impaired renal or hepatic function.
  - Side effects: nausea, vomiting, diarrhea, constipation, cytopenias, and erythema at injection site. Renal function and hepatic function should be monitored.
- Chemotherapy
  - Patients with high-risk MDS, particularly those with RAEB-1 and RAEB-2, have a poor prognosis, with median survival measured in months.
  - Chemotherapy with AML-type regimens (eg, idarubicin plus cytarabine) results in complete remission rates of up to 62% and 3-year disease-free survival rates of about 15%.[9]
  - Other chemotherapy regimens have been investigated but are not likely to be superior to idarubicin plus cytarabine.[10]
  - Therefore, AML-type chemotherapy may be tried in patients with high-risk MDS, particularly those with RAEB-2 who do not have a bone marrow donor.
- Allogeneic hematopoietic cell transplantation (HCT)
  - Allogeneic HCT may be curative in patients with MDS.[11-13]
  - A number of problems are associated with this approach:
    - The majority of patients with MDS are too old to be considered for conventional allogeneic HCT.

The incidence of graft-versus-host disease is high in older adults receiving allogeneic HCT.
    - HLA-matched sibling donors are available for only 25% of patients.
    - Cure rates with HCT are higher in patients with low-risk disease than in those with high-risk disease.
    - Matched unrelated donor and partially mismatched related donor transplants have considerable morbidity.
  - Nonmyeloablative HCT is investigational but offers promise for decreasing toxicity.
- Investigational therapies
  - A number of new drugs have been and continue to be tested in clinical trials in patients with MDS,[14] including thalidomide,[15] decitabine, arsenic trioxide, immunosuppressive drugs, and the thalidomide derivate lenalidomide (Revlimid®). Immunosuppressive drugs may be reasonable to try in patients with the hypocellular variant of MDS.
  - At the time of this writing, the FDA has not approved any of these agents for use in patients with MDS.
- Conclusions
  - In older patients with low-risk disease, management generally consists of observation or supportive care with transfusions and growth factors.
  - In younger patients with high-risk disease and an HLA-identical sibling, allogeneic transplantation may be curative.
  - The newly approved hypomethylating agent azacytidine is superior to supportive care in decreasing transfusion requirements, improving quality of life, and decreasing the rate of progression to AML.

References

1. Brunning RD, Bennett JM, Flandrin G, et al. Myelodysplastic syndromes. In: Jaffe ES, Harris NL, Stein H, Vardiman JW, eds. *Pathology and Genetics of Tumours of Haematopoietic and Lymphoid Tissues*. Lyon: IARC Press; 2001:61-73.

2. Bennett JM, Catovsky D, Daniel MT, et al. Proposals for the classification of the myelodysplastic syndromes. *Br J Haematol.* 1982;51:189-199.
3. Jaffe ES, Harris NL, Stein H, Vardiman JW, eds. *Pathology and Genetics of Tumours of Haematopoietic and Lymphoid Tissues*. Lyon: IARC Press; 2001.
4. Heaney ML, Golde DW. Myelodysplasia. *N Engl J Med.* 1999;340:1649-1660.
5. Greenberg P, Cox C, LeBeau MM, et al. International scoring system for evaluating prognosis in myelodysplastic syndromes. *Blood.* 1997;89:2079-2088.
6. Casadevall N, Durieux P, Dubois S, et al. Health, economic, and quality-of-life effects of erythropoietin and granulocyte colony-stimulating factor for the treatment of myelodysplastic syndromes: a randomized, controlled trial. *Blood.* 2004;104:321-327.
7. Kornblith AB, Herndon JE, 2nd, Silverman LR, et al. Impact of azacytidine on the quality of life of patients with myelodysplastic syndrome treated in a randomized phase III trial: a Cancer and Leukemia Group B study. *J Clin Oncol.* 2002;20:2441-2452.
8. Silverman LR, Demakos EP, Peterson BL, et al. Randomized controlled trial of azacitidine in patients with the myelodysplastic syndrome: a study of the Cancer and Leukemia Group B. *J Clin Oncol.* 2002;20:2429-2440.
9. Anderlini P, Pierce S, Kantarjian H, Estey E. Acute myeloid leukemia-type chemotherapy for myelodysplasia. *J Clin Oncol.* 1996;14:1404-1405.
10. Estey EH, Thall PF, Cortes JE, et al. Comparison of idarubicin + ara-C-, fludarabine + ara-C-, and topotecan + ara-C-based regimens in treatment of newly diagnosed acute myeloid leukemia, refractory anemia with excess blasts in transformation, or refractory anemia with excess blasts. *Blood.* 2001;98:3575-3583.
11. Deeg HJ, Appelbaum FR. Hematopoietic stem cell transplantation in patients with myelodysplastic syndrome. *Leuk Res.* 2000;24:653-663.
12. Deeg HJ, Storer B, Slattery JT, et al. Conditioning with targeted busulfan and cyclophosphamide for hemopoietic stem cell transplantation from related and unrelated donors in patients with myelodysplastic syndrome. *Blood.* 2002; 100:1201-1207.
13. Castro-Malaspina H, Harris RE, Gajewski J, et al. Unrelated donor marrow transplantation for myelodysplastic

syndromes: outcome analysis in 510 transplants facilitated by the National Marrow Donor Program. *Blood.* 2002; 99:1943-1951.

14. Estey EH. Current challenges in therapy of myelodysplastic syndromes. *Curr Opin Hematol.* 2003;10:60-67.
15. Raza A, Meyer P, Dutt D, et al. Thalidomide produces transfusion independence in long-standing refractory anemias of patients with myelodysplastic syndromes. *Blood.* 2001; 98:958-965.

CHAPTER 4

Acute Lymphoblastic Leukemia

Epidemiology

- In the United States, an estimated 3,970 new cases will occur in 2005.[1]
- ALL is the most common leukemia in children but accounts for only 20% of cases of acute leukemia in adults.
- About 80% of cases are of precursor B-cell phenotype.
- 75% of cases of precursor B-ALL occur in children younger than 6 years of age.

Classification

- The FAB classification[2,3] is based on morphology and contains little valuable prognostic implication, so it is not used much anymore. Three categories of ALL are described:
  - L1
    - Greater than 50% of blasts are small.
    - Greater than 75% of blasts have a high nuclear-to-cytoplasmic ratio.
    - Greater than 75% of blasts have up to one small, ill-defined nucleolus.
    - Greater than 75% of blasts have a regular nuclear membrane.
  - L2: the opposite of L1, in that blasts tend to be larger with moderate amounts of cytoplasm and prominent nucleoli
  - L3 (Burkitt): blasts are large, homogenous, and characterized by basophilic cytoplasm with prominent vacuoles
- World Health Organizations (WHO) classification[4,5]
  - Precursor B lymphoblastic leukemia/lymphoma.

    - Distinguished by absence of staining of blasts with myeloperoxidase and characteristic immunophenotype.
    - Immunophenotypic analysis allows identification of three subtypes: early precursor B-ALL, common ALL, and pre-B ALL (Table 4-1).
  - Precursor T lymphoblastic leukemia/lymphoma: distinguished by absence of staining of blasts with myeloperoxidase and characteristic immunophenotype
  - Burkitt lymphoma/leukemia (mature B): distinguished by characteristic morphology of blasts (L3 type), characteristic immunophenotype (expression of surface immunoglobulin and other B-cell markers), and characteristic genetic abnormalities (rearrangements of 8q24)
- ALL versus lymphoblastic lymphoma
  - The distinction between these two entities is somewhat arbitrary and usually does not affect management.
  - In a patient with a lymph node mass and fewer than 25% lymphoblasts in the bone marrow, the term "lymphoblastic lymphoma" is preferred. On the other hand, if 25% or greater of the nucleated cells in the bone marrow are lymphoblasts, the term "acute lymphoblastic leukemia" is preferred.

Pathology

- Morphology[3]
  - Blasts in blood and bone marrow are usually small or medium-sized. They contain scant cytoplasm and moderately condensed or dispersed chromatin. Nucleoli are not as prominent as in AML (Figure 4-1).
  - A cytoplasmic tail, which causes the cell to look like a "hand mirror," may be observed.
  - Auer rods are absent.
- Genetics
  - Principles
    - Acute leukemia, both lymphoblastic and myeloid, begins when a single progenitor cell acquires one or

Table 4-1: Immunologic Classification of B-Lineage ALL

Subtype	CD10	CD19	TdT	Cytoplasmic mu	Surface Ig
Early precursor B-ALL	−	+	+	−	−
Common ALL	+	+	+	−	−
Pre-B ALL	+	+	+	+	−
Mature B-ALL	±	+	−	−	+

ALL, acute lymphoblastic leukemia.

Modified with permission from Devine and Larson. Acute leukemia in adults: recent developments in diagnosis and treatment. *CA Cancer J Clin*. 1994;44:326-352.

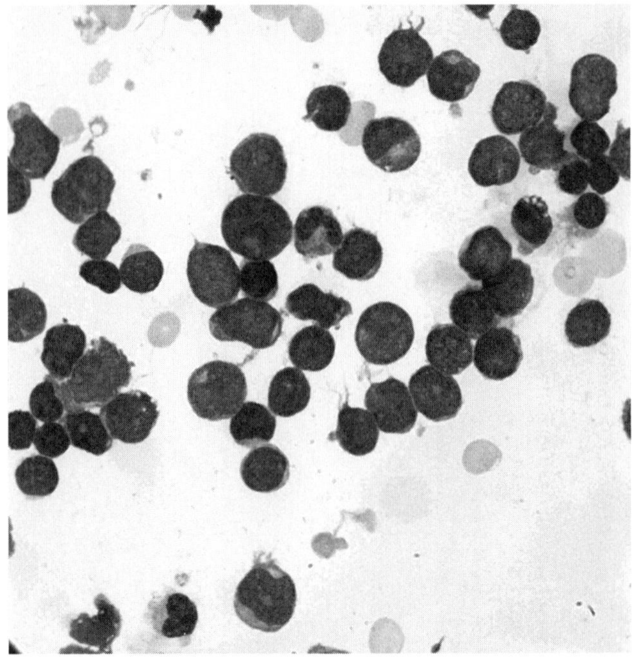

Figure 4-1: Bone marrow aspirate in a patient with acute lymphoblastic leukemia. The blasts are small in size and contain scant cytoplasm.

more genetic mutations that lead to dysregulated growth and impaired differentiation into more mature cells.

- The large majority of cases of ALL are associated with detectable gene mutations in the lymphoblasts.
- Most of these gene mutations are chromosomal translocations, but abnormalities of chromosome numbers (ie, hypodiploidy, hyperdiploidy) occur as well.

- Common abnormalities
  - t(9;22)(q34;q11.2)—Philadelphia chromosome (Ph)
    - More common in adults (25% of cases) than in children (3% of cases)[6]

- Ph is the shortened chromosome 22 that results from the reciprocal translocation between the long arm of chromosome 9 and the long arm of chromosome 22.[7,8]
- As a result of this translocation, the *BCR* (breakpoint cluster region) gene from chromosome 22 is placed next to the *ABL* gene from chromosome 9. This fusion gene results in the expression of BCR-ABL messenger ribonucleic acid (mRNA), which is translated to a functional BCR-ABL protein. This protein is a constitutive tyrosine kinase.[7,8]
- Different breakpoints exist in the *BCR* gene and result in production of either a 190-kd BCR-ABL fusion protein or a 210-kd BCR-ABL fusion protein. These two fusion proteins can be distinguished using PCR methods. In patients with chronic myeloid leukemia (CML), the p210 variant is nearly always present. In adult patients with Ph-positive ALL, 50–75% have the p190 variant, and the rest have the p210 variant.[7,8]
- Confers a poor prognosis due to short duration of remission

- Rearrangements involving 11q23
  - Occur in about 10% of adults with ALL[6]
  - The most common rearrangement involving 11q23 is t(4;11), which results in fusion of the *MLL* gene at 11q23 with *AF4* at 4q21.[7]
  - Confer a poor prognosis
- Hyperdiploid >50 (most cells contain >50 chromosomes)
  - More common in children (25% of cases) than in adults (7% of cases)[6]
  - Confers a favorable prognosis
- t(12;21)(p13;q22)
  - More common in children (22% of cases) than in adults (2% of cases)[6]
  - Requires molecular techniques, such as PCR or FISH, for detection because not detected by standard cytogenetics[7]

    - Results in fusion of *TEL* gene at 12p13 with *AML1* gene at 21q22
    - Confers a favorable prognosis
  - Rearrangements involving 8q24[5]
    - These rearrangements occur in all patients with mature B (Burkitt) ALL.
    - The most common rearrangement is t(8;14), which results in the translocation of the *MYC* gene from chromosome 8 to the immunoglobulin heavy chain region on chromosome 14.
    - Other rearrangements include t(2;8) and t(8;22).
    - These translocations result in the constitutive expression of *MYC*; this expression is thought to be critical in the pathogenesis of mature B ALL.
- Immunophenotype
  - Immunophenotyping allows the distinction between different types (eg, precursor B vs. precursor T) and subtypes of ALL. In addition, immunophenotyping allows the identification of minimally differentiated AML.
  - Immunophenotypic features of the various types of ALL
    - Precursor B-lineage leukemia
      - Almost always positive: terminal deoxynucleotidyl transferase (TdT), HLA-DR, CD19, cytoplasmic CD79a
      - Usually positive: CD10, CD24
      - Occasionally positive: CD20, cytoplasmic CD22 (lineage-specific), CD13, CD33
      - May be further subdivided into early precursor B-ALL, common ALL, and pre-B ALL (see Table 4-1)
    - Precursor T-lineage leukemia
      - Commonly positive: cytoplasmic CD3 (lineage-specific), CD4, CD7, CD8, TdT
      - Variably positive: CD2, CD5, CD10, CD13, CD33, CD79a, CD117
    - Mature B-ALL
      - Always positive: membrane immunoglobulin with light chain restriction

  - Commonly positive: CD10, CD19, CD20, CD22, CD79a
  - Usually negative: CD5, CD23, CD34, TdT
- Blasts of one lineage may express antigens not usually associated with that lineage. These are called "mixed-lineage leukemias." For example, blasts of precursor B lineage may express CD13, an antigen normally associated with the myeloid lineage. This aberrant antigen expression allows detection of a small number of leukemic blasts after treatment, even in patients whose peripheral blood and bone marrow appear morphologically normal.

Prognosis

- Adverse prognostic factors in B-lineage ALL
  - Older age: this is probably a continuous variable, in that the older the patient, the worse the prognosis. Different groups have used different cutoff values between 35 and 60 years.
  - High WBC count: this is probably a continuous variable, in that the higher the WBC count, the worse the prognosis is for achieving and maintaining CR. Different groups have used different cutoff values between 10,000/μL and 30,000/μL.
  - Cytogenetics: t(9;22), t(4;11), −7, trisomy 8
  - Immunophenotype: mature B-ALL has a poor prognosis when treated with conventional ALL regimens. However, with modern regimens designed more specifically for this disease, the prognosis is improved.
  - Delayed time to CR (>4–6 weeks)
- Favorable prognostic factors in T-lineage ALL
  - Mediastinal mass
  - Younger age
  - CD10 antigen expression

Treatment

- Induction
  - Principles
    - There is no single, "standard" induction regimen. Different institutions and cooperative groups have

investigated a variety of induction regimens. Rates of CR and long-term survival have been similar with many of these regimens. Comparing results of different trials is problematic given their sequential, phase II nature. Few randomized, phase III trials have been performed.

- Most induction regimens use several different chemotherapy drugs. Vincristine and prednisone are usually included. Other drugs used include anthracyclines, such as doxorubicin, daunorubicin, cyclophosphamide, and asparaginase.

- Examples of induction regimens (Table 4-2)
  - UCSF 8707[9]
    - Daunorubicin 60 mg/m^2 IV on days 1–3 (and on day 15 if bone marrow on day 14 shows residual leukemia)
    - Vincristine 1.4 mg/m^2 (capped at 2 mg if aged >40 years) IV on days 1, 8, 15, and 22
    - Prednisone 60 mg/m^2 PO on days 1–28
    - Asparaginase 6,000 U/m^2 SC on days 17–28
  - CALGB 9111[10]
    - Daunorubicin 45 mg/m^2 (or 30 mg/m^2 if aged ≥60 years) IV on days 1–3
    - Vincristine 2 mg IV on days 1, 8, 15, and 22
    - Prednisone 60 mg/m^2 PO daily on days 1–21
    - L-asparaginase (*E. coli*) 6,000 IU/m^2 SC/IM on days 5, 8, 11, 15, 18, and 22
    - Cyclophosphamide 1,200 mg/m^2 IV on day 1
  - Hyper-CVAD (MD Anderson regimen)[11]
    - Doxorubicin 50 mg/m^2 IV on day 4
    - Vincristine 2 mg IV on days 4 and 11
    - Dexamethasone 40 mg PO daily on days 1–4 and 11–14
    - Cyclophosphamide 300 mg/m^2 IV every 12 hours on days 1–3
    - Mesna 600 mg/m^2 IVCI over 24 hours daily × 3 days, ending 6 hours after the last dose
  - L20 (Memorial Sloan-Kettering Cancer Center [MSKCC] regimen)

Table 4-2: Comparison of Drugs and Doses Used in Selected ALL Induction Regimens

Drug	UCSF 8707	CALGB 9111	Hyper-CVAD	L20
Daunorubicin	60 mg/m^2 IV on days 1–3	45 mg/m^2 IV on days 1–3	—	—
Doxorubicin	—	—	50 mg/m^2 IV on day 4	60 mg/m^2 IV on day 23; 30 mg/m^2 on day 42
Vincristine	1.4 mg/m^2 IV on days 1, 8, 15, and 22	2 mg IV on days 1, 8, 15, and 22	2 mg IV on days 4 and 11	2 mg/m^2 IV on days 1, 8, 15, 22, and 29
Prednisone	60 mg/m^2 PO daily × 28 days	60 mg/m^2 PO daily × 21 days	—	60 mg/m^2 PO daily × 30 days
Dexamethasone	—	—	40 mg PO on days 1–4 and 11–14	—
Asparaginase	6,000 IU/m^2 SC on days 17–28	6,000 IU/m^2 SC on days 5, 8, 11, 15, 18, and 22	—	—
Cyclophosphamide	—	1,200 mg/m^2 IV on day 1	300 mg/m^2 IV every 12 hours on days 1–3	1,000 mg/m^2 IV on day 5; 600 mg/m^2 IV on day 42

ALL, acute lymphoblastic leukemia; IV, intraveneously; PO, by mouth; SC, subcutaneously.

- Doxorubicin 60 mg/m^2 IV on day 23 and 30 mg/m^2 IV on day 42
- Vincristine 2 mg/m^2 (capped at 4 mg for patients younger than 60 years of age and capped at 2.5 mg for patients older than 60 years of age) IV on days 1, 8, 15, 22, and 19
- Prednisone 60 mg/m^2 PO on days 1–30, then tapered over 10 days
- Cyclophosphamide 1,000 mg/m^2 IV on day 5 and 600 mg/m^2 IV on day 42

- Others: LALA 87,[12] GIMEMA 0288,[13] ECOG 3486,[14] SWOG L10M,[15] GMALL.[16]

- Efficacy of induction regimens (Table 4-3)
  - With modern chemotherapy regimens, the complete remission rate in adult patients with ALL is about 70–90%.
  - However, the 5-year survival rate is only about 25–50%.
  - Although most patients achieve complete remission, the majority of patients relapse and die from their disease.
- Complications of induction
  - Tumor lysis syndrome
  - Infections
  - Cytopenias
    - Neutropenia, anemia, and thrombocytopenia are nearly universal complications of induction and consolidation chemotherapy regimens.
    - The median time to recovery from these cytopenias varies depending on the chemotherapy regimen and the target used to define "recovery," but generally is about 14–21 days.
  - Death: as noted in Table 4-3, up to 10% of patients may die during induction therapy, either as a result of the leukemia itself or from complications of chemotherapy.

- Postremission therapy: consolidation and intensification
  - Principles
    - Patients who achieve CR almost universally relapse without further chemotherapy because of the persistence of minimal residual disease.

Table 4-3: Efficacy of Selected Induction Regimens in ALL

Study	Complete remission (%)	Median survival (mn)	Overall survival	Death during induction (%)
CALGB 9111 (9)	82	23	43% (3 years)	8
UCSF 8707 (8)	93	NR	47% (5 years)	1
Hyper-CVAD (10)	91	35	39% (5 years)	6
LALA 87 (11)	76	NR	27% (10 years)	9

ALL, acute lymphoblastic leukemia; NR, not reported.

    - The aim of postremission therapy is to eliminate minimal residual disease, thereby curing patients of their leukemia.
    - The ideal drug or combination of drugs to use as postremission therapy is unknown. Evaluating the contribution of each individual drug or component of these complex treatment schedules is difficult if not impossible, given the independent, phase II nature of most of the trials.
    - Different cooperative groups have used different regimens, with no regimen clearly being superior in phase II trials.
  - Examples of consolidation/intensification regimens
    - UCSF 8707: alternating courses of high-dose ara-C plus high-dose etoposide, high-dose methotrexate plus 6-mercaptopurine, and the same drugs used in induction (daunorubicin, vincristine, prednisone, and asparaginase)[9]
    - CALGB 9111: two courses of cyclophosphamide, 6-mercaptopurine, cytarabine, vincristine, and asparaginase; one course of doxorubicin, vincristine, dexamethasone, cyclophosphamide, 6-thioguanine, and cytarabine[10]
    - Hyper-CVAD (MD Anderson regimen): alternating cycles of the induction Hyper-CVAD regimen with a regimen containing high-dose methotrexate and high-dose cytarabine[11]
    - L20 (MSKCC regimen): one course of cytarabine plus daunorubicin, one course of cytarabine plus methotrexate, one course of asparaginase, and one course of cyclophosphamide
- Postremission therapy: maintenance
  - Principles
    - Maintenance therapy refers to the use of a prolonged course of outpatient chemotherapy to "maintain" clinical remission.
    - In adult ALL, the use of maintenance therapy has not been proven to be beneficial. Nevertheless, maintenance therapy remains a standard component of most ALL protocols.

        - The optimal drugs and duration of therapy are unknown. Most protocols use methotrexate and 6-mercaptopurine for 2–3 years.
    - Examples of maintenance regimens
        - UCSF 8707: methotrexate 20 mg/m^2 PO weekly and 6-mercaptopurine 75 mg/m^2 PO daily for 30 months[9]
        - CALGB 9111: methotrexate 20 mg/m^2 PO weekly, 6-mercaptopurine 60 mg/m^2 PO daily, vincristine 2 mg IV monthly, and prednisone 60 mg/m^2 PO daily for 5 days every month, all continued until 24 months after diagnosis[10]
        - Hyper-CVAD (MD Anderson regimen): methotrexate 10 mg/m^2 IV daily for 5 days every month, 6-mercaptopurine 1,000 mg/m^2 IV daily for 5 days every month, vincristine 2 mg IV monthly, and prednisone 200 mg PO daily for 5 days every month, all for 2 years[11]
        - L20 (MSKCC regimen): cycles of vincristine, prednisone, doxorubicin, oral methotrexate, oral 6-mercaptopurine, and dactinomycin, alternating with cycles of the same drugs except carmustine and cyclophosphamide instead of doxorubicin, continued for 2 years
- Central nervous system (CNS) prophylaxis and CNS leukemia[17]
    - Principles
        - CNS leukemia is present in fewer than 10% of patients at diagnosis.
        - However, the CNS is a common sanctuary for ALL blasts. As a result, without special attention to CNS prophylaxis, CNS relapse occurs in 20–50% of patients.
        - Because patients with ALL have a high risk of developing CNS leukemia, treatment designed to prevent relapse of leukemia in the CNS, or "CNS prophylaxis," is often administered. CNS prophylaxis lowers the rate of CNS relapse to less than 10%.

- Depending on the protocol, CNS prophylaxis may consist of intrathecal chemotherapy with methotrexate or cytarabine, high doses of systemic methotrexate or cytarabine (which achieve therapeutic levels in the spinal fluid), CNS irradiation, or a combination of the above. The best use of these treatment modalities is not clear. Different cooperative groups and centers have used different combinations of these treatment modalities, but no combination has been definitively proven to be superior to the others.
- Toxicities of CNS prophylaxis include neuropsychiatric sequelae (eg, memory loss, poor concentration, gait unsteadiness), decreased tolerance to systemic chemotherapy, and the development of brain tumors. In order to try to minimize toxicity, many recent protocols have eliminated cranial irradiation.

- Examples of approaches to CNS prophylaxis (Table 4-4)
  - UCSF 8707[9]
    - Cranial irradiation: none
    - Intrathecal chemotherapy: six doses of intrathecal methotrexate (12 mg), the first given at the start of induction. Five subsequent doses are given weekly, beginning with the first course of postremission therapy.
    - High-dose systemic chemotherapy: two courses of high-dose cytarabine and three courses of high-dose methotrexate
    - The rate of CNS relapse in the trial was 3%.
  - CALGB 8811[18]
    - Cranial irradiation: 24 Gy given after three courses of chemotherapy
    - Intrathecal chemotherapy: methotrexate 15 mg given once during both course 2 and course 3 of chemotherapy, then given 5 times during and after cranial irradiation
    - High-dose systemic chemotherapy: none
    - The rate of CNS relapse in the trial was 15%.

Table 4-4: Approaches to CNS Prophylaxis Used in Three Different Protocols

	UCSF 8707	CALGB 8811	Hyper-CVAD
Cranial irradiation	None	24 Gy given after 3 courses of chemotherapy	None
Intrathecal chemotherapy	6 doses of methotrexate 12 mg	7 doses of methotrexate 15 mg	Low-risk patients: 2 doses of methotrexate 12 mg and cytarabine 100 mg High-risk patients: 8 doses of methotrexate 12 mg and cytarabine 100 mg
High-dose systemic therapy	2 courses of high-dose cytarabine; 3 courses of high-dose methotrexate	None	4 courses of high-dose methotrexate and high-dose cytarabine
CNS relapse rate	3%	15%	3%

CNS, central nervous system.

*The MD Anderson Hyper-CVAD protocol is unique in that it classifies patients as low risk or high risk for the development of CNS leukemia. High-risk patients are those with an LDH of >600 U/L, a proliferative index (% S-phase + G_2M-phase) of ≥14%, or mature B-ALL. Low-risk patients are those with none of these three characteristics.

- Hyper-CVAD (MD Anderson regimen)[11]
  - Patients risk-stratified and treated according to risk
    - High risk
      - Lactate dehydrogenase (LDH) greater than 600 U/L, or
      - Proliferative index (% S-phase + G_2M-phase) 14% or more, or
      - Mature B-ALL
    - Low risk: normal LDH and low proliferative index
  - Cranial irradiation: none
  - Intrathecal chemotherapy: methotrexate 12 mg on day 2 and cytarabine 100 mg on day 8 of each of eight cycles in high-risk patients and of each of two cycles in low-risk patients
  - High-dose systemic therapy: four courses of high-dose methotrexate and high-dose cytarabine
  - The rate of CNS relapse in the trial was 3%.
- Clinical features of CNS leukemia
  - Cranial neuropathies
  - Increased intracranial pressure: headaches, nausea, vomiting, lethargy, papilledema
- Treatment of CNS leukemia
  - Like CNS prophylaxis, the treatment of CNS leukemia is not standardized.
  - Patients whose initial presentation is with CNS leukemia usually receive intensified (eg, twice weekly) intrathecal chemotherapy during systemic induction chemotherapy. Cranial irradiation may be administered after achievement of bone marrow remission.
  - Patients who develop relapse in the CNS without simultaneous bone marrow relapse usually develop bone marrow relapse unless a change in systemic therapy occurs. Therefore, isolated CNS relapse is usually treated with systemic reinduction chemotherapy and intrathecal chemotherapy, followed by cranial irradiation.

- Autologous and allogeneic HCT
  - Principles
    - Involves use of high-dose, myeloablative chemotherapy with or without total body radiation, followed by infusion of hematopoietic cells. The infused hematopoietic cells reconstitute the bone marrow, thereby preventing death from myeloablation.
    - In autologous HCT, hematopoietic stem cells are collected from the patient's own peripheral blood or bone marrow. In allogeneic HCT, hematopoietic stem cells are collected from the peripheral blood or bone marrow of a HLA-matched donor—either a sibling or an unrelated person.
    - Allogeneic HCT may be complicated by graft-versus-host disease, in which donor cells recognize normal host cells as foreign and cause skin lesions, liver disease, and diarrhea.
    - The risk of mortality within 100 days of allogeneic HCT for acute leukemia is approximately 20–30%. Causes of mortality include graft-versus-host disease, infections, and regimen-related toxicity.
    - Allogeneic HCT in ALL may be associated with a "graft-versus-leukemia effect." This refers to the ability of transplanted donor cells to attack residual leukemia cells in the recipient. Evidence for this graft-versus-leukemia effect include a lower rate of relapse in patients who develop graft-versus-host disease after transplantation and the achievement of CRs by donor lymphocyte infusions in patients who experience relapse after transplantation.[19-20]
    - The role of autologous HCT in the treatment of ALL is unclear. No survival benefit has been demonstrated.
    - Allogeneic HCT is routinely used in patients with high-risk disease, such as those with t(4;11) or t(9;22), in first CR, and in other patients who experience relapse but achieve a second complete remission.

  - The ideal preparative regimen for transplantation is not known. Most protocols have used total body irradiation with chemotherapy drugs such as cyclophosphamide, etoposide, and others.
  - Most protocols have used bone marrow as the source of hematopoietic stem cells. Recently, use of peripheral blood stem cells has become more common in many centers.
- Transplantation in first CR
  - Autologous HCT versus postremission chemotherapy
    - In the French LALA 87 protocol, 191 patients younger than 50 years of age who lacked an HLA-matched sibling donor but were in complete remission were randomized to receive consolidation chemotherapy followed by maintenance chemotherapy or consolidation chemotherapy followed by autologous HCT. The percentage of patients alive at 10 years was similar (about 30%) in both arms.[12] One notable feature of this study is that many patients in the transplantation arm experienced relapse during consolidation therapy, raising the question of whether HCT earlier in remission would provide benefit.[22]
  - Autologous versus allogeneic HCT
    - Attal et al treated 120 adults with ALL in first CR using "genetic randomization." Patients with an HLA-identical sibling received allogeneic HCT; the rest received autologous HCT. The rate of disease-free survival at 3 years was higher in the allogeneic HCT group than in the autologous HCT group (68% vs. 28%, respectively, $P < .001$).[23] Overall survival was not reported.
    - In the French LALA 87 protocol, 257 adults with ALL achieved CR. Patients with an HLA-identical sibling received allogeneic HCT; the rest received 3 months of consolidation chemotherapy and were then randomized to receive more chemotherapy or autologous HCT.

Allogeneic HCT improved both disease-free and 10-year overall survival rates. However, on subset analysis, the benefit was restricted to high-risk patients.[12,24]

- Several other randomized and retrospective studies have attempted to evaluate the role of allogeneic HCT in patients with ALL in first remission. In general, these trials have demonstrated that allogeneic HCT lowers the relapse rate but increases treatment-related mortality. These effects tend to offset one another in standard-risk patients, resulting in similar long-term outcomes compared with conventional chemotherapy. However, in high-risk patients, allogeneic HCT in first remission improves overall survival.
- An ongoing trial of ECOG and the Medical Research Council in Britain is comparing conventional chemotherapy, autologous HCT, and allogeneic HCT for patients in first CR. Preliminary results indicate improved 5-year event-free survival in patients receiving allogeneic HCT. Overall survival has not been reported. The trial is still ongoing.[25]
- The Southwest Oncology Group is comparing conventional chemotherapy and allogeneic HCT for patients in first CR.

■ In summary, in standard-risk patients, transplantation in first CR probably improves event-free survival, although no convincing overall survival benefit has been demonstrated. Therefore, this approach is generally considered investigational. On the other hand, allogeneic HCT in first CR is the preferred treatment for high-risk patients, such as those with t(9;22) or t(4;11), with HLA-matched donors.

- Transplantation in second or greater remission
  - ■ Although many patients with relapsed ALL achieve a second remission following salvage chemotherapy, the remission duration is usually short, and

long-term disease-free survival is rare. Allogeneic HCT offers these patients the best chance of cure. Therefore, if an HLA-matched sibling donor is available, allogeneic HCT should be performed.

- In patients with relapsed disease undergoing autologous HCT, the long-term disease-free survival rate is approximately 20–25%. These outcomes appear favorable compared with those achieved with conventional chemotherapy. However, randomized trials have not been performed, so this approach remains investigational.

- Treatment of specific populations
  - Ph-positive ALL
    - CR rates after induction chemotherapy in patients with Ph-positive ALL are similar, if slightly inferior, to those in patients with Ph-negative disease (60–80%). However, when conventional chemotherapy regimens are used, the duration of remission and the event-free survival rates (about 10%) in patients with Ph-positive disease are lower than those in patients with Ph-negative disease.
    - Allogeneic HCT in first CR has resulted in long-term survival rates of greater than 35% in several series.
    - Therefore, allogeneic HCT in first CR is the preferred treatment in Ph-positive patients with an HLA-identical sibling donor.
    - In a phase II study of 56 patients with relapsed or refractory Ph-positive ALL, imatinib mesylate (Gleevec®), an inhibitor of the BCR-ABL tyrosine kinase, induced complete hematologic responses in 19%, complete bone marrow responses in 10%, and complete cytogenetic responses in 17%. Unfortunately, the median time to progression was only 2.2 months, and the median overall survival was only 4.9 months, indicating the rapid development of resistance to imatinib in nearly all cases.[26]
    - Current studies are investigating the efficacy and toxicity of adding imatinib earlier in the course of treatment for patients with Ph-positive ALL.[27]

- Mature B (Burkitt-type) ALL
  - Epidemiology
    - A rare disease, accounting for less than 5% of adult ALL
    - Associated with the acquired immunodeficiency syndrome
  - Morphology: FAB-L3 morphology
  - Immunophenotype: monoclonal surface immunoglobulin present
  - Genetics: usually t(8;14) or variants t(8;22) and t(2;8)
  - Clinical features: high rate of CNS involvement, hepatomegaly, splenomegaly, lymphadenopathy, and high levels of uric acid and LDH
  - Prognosis
    - Poor when conventional ALL regimens are used (CR rate <40%, long-term survival rare)
    - Much better when dose-intensive regimens containing methotrexate, cytarabine, and cyclophosphamide are used (CR rate 63–86%, long-term survival >45%)
  - Treatment
    - Should consist of a dose-intense regimen containing methotrexate, cytarabine, and cyclophosphamide[11,28,29]
    - CNS prophylaxis must be included.
- T-cell ALL
  - Epidemiology
    - 15–25% of adult ALL
    - More common in young males
  - Clinical features: often have increased WBC count and mediastinal mass
  - Prognosis: favorable in adults with modern regimens (although unfavorable in children)
  - Treatment: same as conventional ALL regimens. Some hypothesize that the incorporation of cyclophosphamide, cytarabine, and asparaginase in induction and consolidation phases of treatment has led to improved outcomes in patients with T-cell ALL.

- Elderly patients
  - Patients older than 60 years of age with ALL have a poor prognosis. Reasons for the poor prognosis probably include a higher frequency of adverse cytogenetics, a lower frequency of T-cell ALL, and poor tolerance of chemotherapy given comorbid conditions.
  - In otherwise healthy, elderly patients with ALL, conventional ALL regimens may be used. Less toxic regimens can be considered in patients with a poor performance status due to comorbid conditions.

- Relapsed or refractory disease
  - As described earlier, many patients with relapsed ALL (40–60%) achieve a second remission following salvage chemotherapy. However, the remission duration is usually short, and long-term disease-free survival is rare.
  - A variety of phase II studies have investigated different chemotherapy regimens designed to induce remission in the relapsed setting. Agents used have included vincristine, steroids, anthracyclines, asparaginase, methotrexate, and cytarabine. Imatinib mesylate has been studied in Ph-positive patients.
  - Of these regimens, none can be considered "standard." The choice of regimen depends largely on the patient's prior therapy and duration of previous remission.
  - In general, patients with relapsed ALL should undergo allogeneic HCT if a suitable donor is available. If relapse occurs after a durable remission, salvage chemotherapy is usually given before transplantation in an attempt to achieve second CR.

References

1. Jemal A, Murray T, Ward E, et al. Cancer statistics, 2005. *CA Cancer J Clin.* 2005;55:10-30.
2. Bennett JM, Catovsky D, Daniel MT, et al. The morphological classification of acute lymphoblastic leukaemia: concordance among observers and clinical correlations. *Br J Haematol.* 1981;47:553-561.

3. Scheinberg DA, Maslak P, Weiss M. Acute leukemias. In: DeVita VT Jr, Hellman S, Rosenberg SA, eds. *Cancer: Principles & Practice of Oncology*. 6th ed. Philadelphia, PA: Lippincott Williams & Wilkins; 2001:2404-2433.
4. Brunning RD, Borowitz M, Matutes E, et al. Precursor B-cell and T-cell neoplasms. In: Jaffe ES, Harris NL, Stein H, Vardiman JW, eds. *Pathology and Genetics of Tumours of Haematopoietic and Lymphoid Tissues*. Lyon: IARC Press; 2001:109-117.
5. Diebold J, Jaffe ES, Raphael M, Warnke RA. Burkitt lymphoma. In: Jaffe ES, Harris NL, Stein H, Vardiman JW, eds. *Pathology and Genetics of Tumours of Haematopoietic and Lymphoid Tissues*. Lyon: IARC Press; 2001:109-117.
6. Pui CH, Relling MV, Downing JR. Acute lymphoblastic leukemia. *N Engl J Med*. 2004;350:1535-1548.
7. Faderl S, Kantarjian HM, Talpaz M, Estrov Z. Clinical significance of cytogenetic abnormalities in adult acute lymphoblastic leukemia. *Blood*. 1998;91:3995-4019.
8. Radich JP. Philadelphia chromosome-positive acute lymphocytic leukemia. *Hematol Oncol Clin North Am*. 2001;15:21-36.
9. Linker C, Damon L, Ries C, Navarro W. Intensified and shortened cyclical chemotherapy for adult acute lymphoblastic leukemia. *J Clin Oncol*. 2002;20:2464-2471.
10. Larson RA, Dodge RK, Linker CA, et al. A randomized controlled trial of filgrastim during remission induction and consolidation chemotherapy for adults with acute lymphoblastic leukemia: CALGB study 9111. *Blood*. 1998; 92:1556-1564.
11. Kantarjian HM, O'Brien S, Smith TL, et al. Results of treatment with hyper-CVAD, a dose-intensive regimen, in adult acute lymphocytic leukemia. *J Clin Oncol*. 2000;18:547-561.
12. Thiebaut A, Vernant JP, Degos L, et al. Adult acute lymphocytic leukemia study testing chemotherapy and autologous and allogeneic transplantation. A follow-up report of the French protocol LALA 87. *Hematol Oncol Clin North Am*. 2000;14:1353-1366.
13. Annino L, Vegna ML, Camera A, et al. Treatment of adult acute lymphoblastic leukemia (ALL): long-term follow-up of the GIMEMA ALL 0288 randomized study. *Blood*. 2002;99:863-871.

14. Wiernik PH, Cassileth PA, Leong T, et al. A randomized trial of induction therapy (daunorubicin, vincristine, prednisone versus daunorubicin, vincristine, prednisone, cytarabine and 6-thioguanine) in adult acute lymphoblastic leukemia with long-term follow-up: an Eastern Cooperative Oncology Group Study (E3486). *Leuk Lymphoma.* 2003;44:1515-1521.
15. Petersdorf SH, Kopecky KJ, Head DR, et al. Comparison of the L10M consolidation regimen to an alternative regimen including escalating methotrexate/L-asparaginase for adult acute lymphoblastic leukemia: a Southwest Oncology Group Study. *Leukemia.* 2001;15:208-216.
16. Gokbuget N, Hoelzer D, Arnold R, et al. Treatment of adult ALL according to protocols of the German Multicenter Study Group for Adult ALL (GMALL). *Hematol Oncol Clin North Am.* 2000;14:1307-1325.
17. Cortes J. Central nervous system involvement in adult acute lymphocytic leukemia. *Hematol Oncol Clin North Am.* 2001;15:145-162.
18. Larson RA, Dodge RK, Burns CP, et al. A five-drug remission induction regimen with intensive consolidation for adults with acute lymphoblastic leukemia: Cancer and Leukemia Group B study 8811. *Blood.* 1995;85:2025-2037.
19. Ringden O, Hermans J, Labopin M, Apperley J, Gorin NC, Gratwohl A. The highest leukaemia-free survival after allogeneic bone marrow transplantation is seen in patients with grade I acute graft-versus-host disease. Acute and Chronic Leukaemia Working Parties of the European Group for Blood and Marrow Transplantation (EBMT). *Leuk Lymphoma.* 1996;24:71-79.
20. Cornelissen JJ, Carston M, Kollman C, et al. Unrelated marrow transplantation for adult patients with poor-risk acute lymphoblastic leukemia: strong graft-versus-leukemia effect and risk factors determining outcome. *Blood.* 2001;97:1572-1577.
21. Kiehl MG, Kraut L, Schwerdtfeger R, et al. Outcome of allogeneic hematopoietic stem-cell transplantation in adult patients with acute lymphoblastic leukemia: no difference in related compared with unrelated transplant in first complete remission. *J Clin Oncol.* 2004;22:2816-2825.
22. Martin TG, Linker CA. Autologous stem cell transplantation for acute lymphocytic leukemia in adults. *Hematol Oncol Clin North Am.* 2001;15:121-143.

23. Attal M, Blaise D, Marit G, et al. Consolidation treatment of adult acute lymphoblastic leukemia: a prospective, randomized trial comparing allogeneic versus autologous bone marrow transplantation and testing the impact of recombinant interleukin-2 after autologous bone marrow transplantation. BGMT Group. *Blood.* 1995;86:1619-1628.
24. Sebban C, Lepage E, Vernant JP, et al. Allogeneic bone marrow transplantation in adult acute lymphoblastic leukemia in first complete remission: a comparative study. French Group of Therapy of Adult Acute Lymphoblastic Leukemia. *J Clin Oncol.* 1994;12:2580-2587.
25. Rowe JM, Richards SM, Burnett AK, et al. Favorable results of allogeneic bone marrow transplantation (BMT) for adults with Philadelphia (Ph)-chromosome-negative acute lymphoblastic leukemia (ALL) in first complete remission (CR): results from the International ALL Trial (MRC UKALL XII/ECOG E2993) [abstract]. *Blood.* 2001;98: 481a. Abstract 2009.
26. Ottmann OG, Druker BJ, Sawyers CL, et al. A phase 2 study of imatinib in patients with relapsed or refractory Philadelphia chromosome-positive acute lymphoid leukemias. *Blood.* 2002;100:1965-1971.
26. Thomas DA, Faderl S, Cortes J, et al. Treatment of Philadelphia chromosome-positive acute lymphocytic leukemia with hyper-CVAD and imatinib mesylate. *Blood.* 2004;103:4396-4407.
27. Soussain C, Patte C, Ostronoff M, et al. Small noncleaved cell lymphoma and leukemia in adults. A retrospective study of 65 adults treated with the LMB pediatric protocols. *Blood.* 1995;85:664-674.
28. Hoelzer D, Ludwig WD, Thiel E, et al. Improved outcome in adult B-cell acute lymphoblastic leukemia. *Blood.* 1996;87:495-508.

CHAPTER 5

Chronic Lymphocytic Leukemia

Definition

- Chronic lymphocytic leukemia (CLL) is a neoplasm of B lymphocytes that accumulate in the blood, bone marrow, lymph nodes, and spleen.[1,2]
- CLL and small lymphocytic lymphoma (SLL) are essentially the same disease. The term SLL is generally used in cases in which lymph node morphology and immunophenotype are characteristic of CLL but the blood and marrow do not contain malignant lymphocytes.

Epidemiology

- In the United States, an estimated 9,730 new cases will occur in 2005.[3]
- Median age at diagnosis is 65 years; only 10% of cases occur in patients under age 50 years.[1]
- M:F = 2:1[2]

Pathology

- Morphology[2]
  - Typically, the malignant lymphocytes in the blood and bone marrow are small, mature-appearing lymphocytes (Figure 5-1). Chromatin is clumped, cytoplasm is scant, and nucleoli are not seen.
  - In some cases, however, the lymphocytes may be larger and more atypical.
  - "Smudge" cells are a characteristic but nonspecific feature.
  - Bone marrow involvement is often classified as nodular, interstitial, or diffuse, with the diffuse pattern usually reflecting more advanced disease (Figure 5-2).

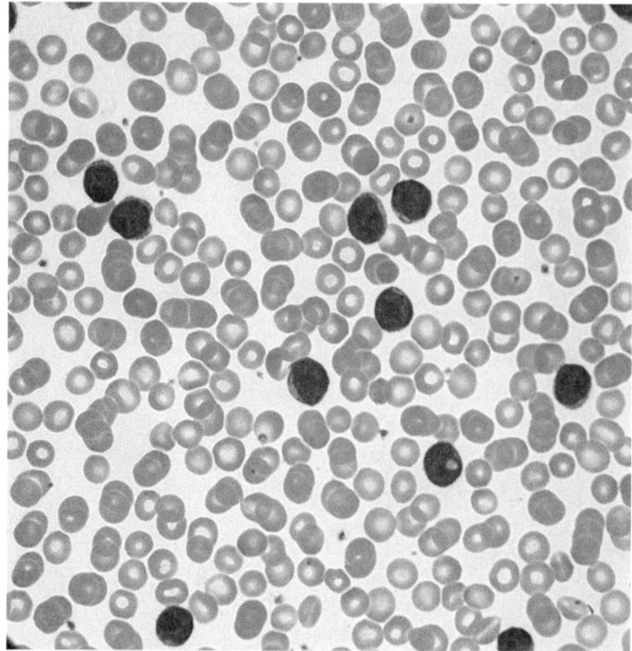

Figure 5-1: Peripheral blood smear of a patient with chronic lymphocytic leukemia. There is an increased number of small- and medium-sized mature-appearing lymphocytes.

- Lymph node architecture is effaced by small, mature lymphocytes.

■ Genetics
- Immunoglobulin V_H genes[4-6]
  - In lymphocytes, germline gene segments called V_H, D, and J_H rearrange to form a gene that encodes the variable region of the heavy chain of the immunoglobulin molecule.
  - Immunoglobulin V_H genes may be either mutated, defined as having greater than 2% somatic mutation compared with the nearest germline V_H gene, or unmutated, defined as having 98% or greater sequence homology with the nearest germline V_H gene.
  - Because somatic mutations in V_H gene segments typically occur in antigen-stimulated B-cells,

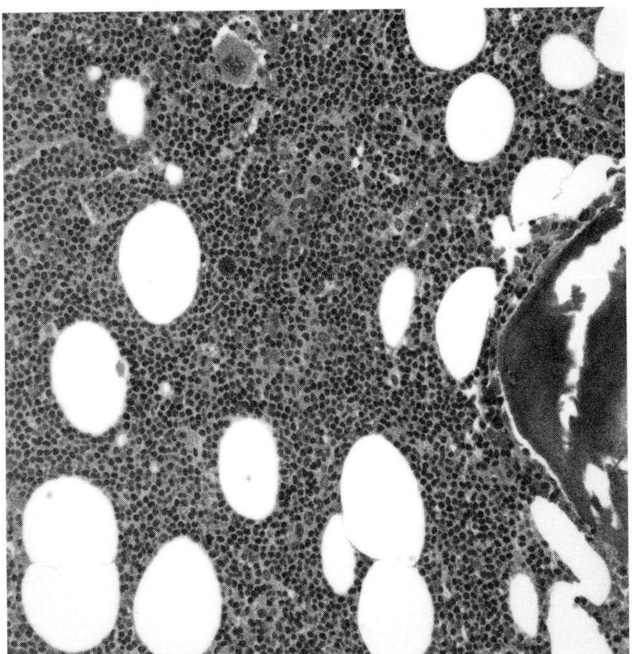

Figure 5-2: Bone marrow biopsy of a patient with chronic lymphocytic leukemia. There is diffuse infiltration of the marrow with mature lymphocytes.

mutated V_H genes in CLL cells indicate that the leukemia arose from memory B-cells, whereas unmutated V_H genes in CLL cells indicate that the leukemia arose from naïve B-cells.

- These differences have prognostic implications, as described below.

- Cytogenetic abnormalities
  - Although CLL cells usually contain genetic abnormalities, the low mitotic activity of CLL cells *in vitro* limits the effectiveness of conventional cytogenetic analysis.
  - With conventional karyotyping, clonal genetic mutations can be detected in approximately 50% of cases.[7]

    - However, when FISH analysis is used, clonal genetic mutations can be detected in about 80% of cases.[8]
    - Common abnormalities include deletions of 13q14, 11q22-23, 6q21, and 17p13 (p53 locus), and trisomy 12.
    - Deletions of 17p13 and 11q22-23 have adverse prognostic implications.[8]
- Immunophenotype
  - CLL cells have a characteristic immunophenotype. In a patient with an absolute lymphocytosis in the peripheral blood, flow cytometry can be used to diagnose or exclude CLL.
  - CD5, CD11c (weak), CD19, CD20 (weak), CD22 (weak), CD23, CD43, CD79a, and surface immunoglobulin (weak) are usually expressed.
  - CD10, cyclin D1, and FMC7 are usually negative.
  - Other B-cell leukemias and lymphomas may produce lymphocytosis and thereby mimic CLL. Immunophenotyping is useful in distinguishing between these disease entities (Table 5-1).
    - In B-cell prolymphocytic leukemia (as in CLL), CD19, CD20, CD22, and CD79a are usually expressed. However, in contrast to CLL, CD5 is expressed in only one third of cases, and CD23 is

Table 5-1: Distinguishing Immunotypic Features of Selected Mature B-Cell Neoplasms

Disease	CD5	CD23	FMC7	sIg
Chronic lymphocytic leukemia	+	+	–	Weak
Mantle cell lymphoma	+	–	+	Strong
Prolymphocytic leukemia	–(2/3)	–	+	Strong

sIg, surface immunoglobulin.

typically not expressed, FMC7 is usually expressed, and surface immunoglobulin is usually strongly expressed.

- In mantle cell lymphoma (as in CLL), CD5, CD19, and CD20 are usually expressed. However, in contrast to CLL, CD23 is usually not expressed, FMC7 is usually expressed, and cyclin D1 is expressed in virtually all cases. Expression of cyclin D1 should be assessed in all B-cell lymphomas that are CD5+ and CD23−.

Clinical Features

- Symptoms
  - Many patients are asymptomatic at presentation, and the diagnosis is made when lymphocytosis is noted on a CBC performed for other reasons.
  - Fatigue and weight loss may occur.
  - Infections are common.
- Signs
  - Lymphadenopathy, often generalized
  - Splenomegaly, hepatomegaly
- Laboratory findings
  - Leukocytosis, lymphocytosis
  - Anemia and thrombocytopenia occur in later stages of the disease.
  - Monoclonal gammopathy and hypogammaglobulinemia may occur.
- Complications[1]
  - Autoimmune complications
    - Positive direct antiglobulin test
    - Autoimmune hemolytic anemia
    - Immune thrombocytopenic purpura
    - Pure red cell aplasia
  - Hypogammaglobulinemia
  - Infections: the risk of bacterial, viral, fungal, and parasitic infections is increased
  - Transformation to diffuse large cell lymphoma (ie, Richter's transformation) occurs in 3–5% of cases.

Diagnostic Evaluation

- History and physical exam
- CBC, metabolic panel, lactate dehydrogenase (LDH), uric acid
- Peripheral blood flow cytometry
- CT scan of the chest, abdomen, and pelvis is optional but may be useful to evaluate the extent of lymphadenopathy.
- Bone marrow examination is optional at the time of diagnosis, particularly if the diagnosis is clear and no immediate treatment is planned. Bone marrow examination is often performed prior to the initiation of therapy and monitored thereafter to assess remission status.

Staging

- Two staging systems are commonly used in CLL: the Rai system[9] and the Binet system[10] (Table 5-2).

Table 5-2: Staging Systems Used for CLL

Staging system	Stage	Clinical features
Rai		
Low risk	0	Lymphocytosis
Intermediate risk	I	Lymphadenopathy
Intermediate risk	II	Hepatomegaly or splenomegaly
High risk	III	Anemia (Hg <11 g/dL)
High risk	IV	Thrombocytopenia (<100,000/mm^3)
Binet		
Low risk	A	No anemia, no thrombocytopenia, <3 node-bearing areas enlarged
Intermediate risk	B	No anemia, no thrombocytopenia, ≥3 node-bearing areas enlarged
High risk	C	Anemia (Hg <10 g/dL) and/or thrombocytopenia

CLL, chronic lymphocytic leukemia.

Modified with permission from Rozman and Montserrat. Chronic lymphocytic leukemia. *N Engl J Med.* 1995;333:1052-1057.

- Because both systems are commonly used, the author recommends that the practicing oncologist be familiar with both.

Prognosis

- Adverse prognostic factors
  - Diffuse infiltration of bone marrow
  - Lymphocyte doubling time 12 months or less
  - Advanced stage
  - Deletion of 17p13 or of 11q22-23[8]
  - Unmutated V_H genes[5]
  - Expression of CD38 on leukemia cells[11]
  - Expression of ZAP-70 in lymphocytes[12]
- Survival by stage[1]
  - In patients with low-risk (Rai stage 0 or Binet stage A) disease, the median survival exceeds 10 years.
  - In patients with intermediate-risk (Rai stage I or II, or Binet stage B) disease, the median survival is between 5 and 8 years.
  - In patients with high-risk (Rai stage III–IV or Binet stage C) disease, the median survival is between 2 and 3 years.

Treatment

- Principles
  - There is no curative therapy.
  - Patients with early and stable disease may survive as long as healthy subjects of the same age.
  - Treatment of asymptomatic patients in the early stages of disease with chlorambucil does not improve survival.[13]
  - Indications for treatment
    - Symptoms from lymphadenopathy or splenomegaly
    - Anemia or thrombocytopenia
    - Rapid lymphocyte doubling time (controversial)
    - Transformation to large cell lymphoma or prolymphocytic leukemia
    - Autoimmune complications
  - In patients without any of the indications for treatment, observation alone is reasonable.

- Single-agent therapy
  - Chlorambucil
    - Mechanism: an alkylating agent
    - Efficacy
      - Responses occur in approximately 35–40% of patients, and CRs occur in approximately 4% of patients.[14]
      - Often given with prednisone
    - Dose: several options exist. The optimal dosing regimen is unknown.
      - 40 mg/m^2, or 0.8 mg/kg, PO once every 28 days[14]
      - 0.3 mg/kg PO daily for 5 days every month[13]
      - 20–30 mg/m^2, or 0.4–0.8 mg/kg, PO every 2 weeks[15]
      - 4–8 mg/m^2, or 0.08–0.1 mg/kg, PO daily[13]
    - Side effects: cytopenias, nausea and vomiting, infertility, seizures, hepatotoxicity, and others
  - Fludarabine
    - Mechanism
      - A nucleoside analog
      - Converted inside cells to the active metabolite 2-fluoro-ara-ATP, which inhibits DNA synthesis and repairs RNA synthesis
    - Efficacy
      - Responses occur in approximately 60–65% of patients, and CRs occur in approximately 20% of patients. The median duration of response is approximately 2 years.[14]
      - In a randomized trial comparing fludarabine with chlorambucil, fludarabine therapy resulted in a significant improvement in response rate and median time to progression but no change in overall survival.[14]
    - Dose
      - 25 mg/m^2 IV daily for 5 days, repeated every 28 days for up to six cycles.
      - In elderly patients or in those with a poor performance status, therapy for a shorter number of days (eg, 3) may be considered.

    - The optimal number of cycles is unknown. Six cycles of therapy is commonly used. It is unknown whether treatment with additional cycles provides clinical benefit in cases in which CR is achieved after fewer than six cycles.
    - Treatment with allopurinol before and during the initial cycle of therapy is recommended to prevent tumor lysis syndrome.
    - Prophylaxis with antibacterial, antiviral, and antifungal antibiotics can be considered but has not been proven to be effective.
  - Side effects: myelosuppression, prolonged lymphopenia, immune suppression and opportunistic infections, neurotoxicity, tumor lysis syndrome, and autoimmune hemolytic anemia
- Rituximab (Rituxan®)
  - Mechanism: a chimeric monoclonal antibody directed at the CD20 antigen
  - Efficacy
    - As a single agent, rituximab has modest activity in CLL.
    - In a dose-escalation study including 40 patients with fludarabine-refractory CLL and 10 with other mature B-cell leukemias, the overall response rate was 36%, with no CRs. The response rate was dose related.[16]
- Alemtuzumab (Campath-1H)
  - Mechanism: a humanized monoclonal antibody directed at the CD52 antigen
  - Efficacy
    - In a trial of 93 patients whose disease had relapsed after or was refractory to fludarabine, treatment with alemtuzumab resulted in an overall response rate of 33% and a CR rate of 2%. The median time to response was 1.5 months.[17] Based on these data, alemtuzumab was approved by the FDA in May 2001 for the treatment of patients with CLL previously treated with alkylating agents and fludarabine.

- Dose and administration
  - The initial dose of alemtuzumab is 3 mg IV over 2 hours daily. Once infusion reactions are well tolerated, the daily dose is increased to 10 mg. When the 10 mg dose is well tolerated, the dose is increased to 30 mg given three times weekly for a maximum of 12 weeks.
  - Acetaminophen 650 mg and diphenhydramine 50 mg should be administered before each treatment to help minimize infusion-related reactions. Patients who develop severe infusion-related reactions may be pretreated with corticosteroids (eg, hydrocortisone 200 mg) and/or meperidine.
  - Antipneumocystis prophylaxis (eg, trimethoprim-sulfamethoxazole 160 mg/800 mg twice daily three times weekly) and antiviral prophylaxis (eg, famciclovir 250 mg twice daily) should be administered because of the risk of opportunistic infections. These antibiotics should be continued for 2 months after completion of alemtuzumab therapy or until the CD4 count rises above 200/μL, whichever occurs later.
  - SC administration has the theoretical advantage of avoiding infusion-related reactions and is under investigation.
- Side effects
  - Infusion-related reactions: rigors, fevers, dyspnea, hypotension, nausea, vomiting, and skin rash are common
  - Cytopenias
  - Infections
    - Alemtuzumab causes depletion of $CD4^+$ and $CD8^+$ T cells, $CD19^+$ B cells, and $CD52^+$ cells, resulting in prolonged immunosuppression that can last up to 18 months and cause opportunistic infections with bacterial, viral, fungal, and protozoal organisms.
    - Antibiotic prophylaxis as described above is mandatory in patients receiving alemtuzumab.

- Others: cyclophosphamide, corticosteroids, and other nucleoside analogs, such as pentostatin and cladribine, also have activity in CLL and may be used in various settings.
- Combination therapy
  - In one trial, the combination of fludarabine and chlorambucil was excessively toxic and no more effective than single-agent therapy.[14]
  - However, other combination chemotherapy regimens have been reported to be effective in phase II trials (eg, fludarabine plus cyclophosphamide,[18] fludarabine plus rituximab,[19] the combination of all three drugs[20,21]).
  - Phase III trials are ongoing.
- Summary
  - In healthy patients deemed fit enough to tolerate fludarabine, most physicians consider single-agent fludarabine to be standard therapy. Combination therapy may also be considered, although a survival benefit has not been demonstrated in randomized trials.
  - In elderly or less fit patients, single-agent chlorambucil is often recommended because it is less toxic and easier to administer than fludarabine. Alternatively, 3-day courses of fludarabine may be used.
  - Alemtuzumab is generally used in the setting of relapse.

Other Considerations in the Management of Patients with CLL

- Splenectomy: useful in cases of symptomatic splenomegaly or hypersplenism in which the disease is refractory to chemotherapy
- Radiation therapy
  - May be considered for palliation of bulky lymph node masses, symptomatic splenomegaly, and hypersplenism
  - Radiation is particularly useful when the disease is refractory to chemotherapy.
- HCT: several centers have reported results of treatment with autologous and allogeneic HCT in patients with

relapsed CLL. Transplantation is still considered investigational in this disease. In young patients with refractory disease, referral to a transplant center should be considered.

- Treatment of hypogammaglobulinemia and prevention of infections
  - In a study of patients with CLL with either hypogammaglobulinemia or a history of infection, treatment with IV immunoglobulin (IVIG) 400 mg/kg every 3 weeks for 1 year reduced the risk of bacterial infections but did not improve survival.[22]
  - Although IVIG is not needed in the majority of CLL patients, its use can be considered in patients with recurrent bacterial infections.
- Treatment of autoimmune complications
  - Autoimmune phenomena, particularly thrombocytopenia and hemolytic anemia, can be life-threatening complications of CLL.
  - The primary initial approach to the management of these conditions is corticosteroid therapy. Chlorambucil may be added to control the underlying CLL. Fludarabine is often avoided in patients with a history of autoimmune hemolytic anemia because of the drug's propensity to exacerbate hemolysis.[23]
  - Other modalities commonly used in the management of autoimmune cytopenias, including IVIG and splenectomy, may also be useful.
- Growth factors
  - Erythropoietin therapy may improve the hemoglobin concentration in patients with Coombs'-negative anemia.
  - Some physicians use G-CSF, pegfilgrastim, or GM-CSF in patients with CLL who develop neutropenia after chemotherapy. However, as suggested in guidelines published by the American Society of Clinical Oncology, reduction of chemotherapy doses may be more appropriate to prevent repeated episodes of neutropenia in patients with incurable malignancies such as CLL.[24]

References

1. Rozman C, Montserrat E. Chronic lymphocytic leukemia. *N Engl J Med.* 1995;333:1052-1057.
2. Müller-Hermelink HK, Catovsky D, Montserrat E, Harris NL. Chronic lymphocytic leukemia/small lymphocytic lymphoma. In: Jaffe ES, Harris NL, Stein H, Vardiman JW, eds. *Pathology and Genetics of Tumours of Haematopoietic and Lymphoid Tissues*. Lyon: IARC Press; 2001:127-130.
3. Jemal A, Murray T, Ward E, et al. Cancer statistics, 2005. *CA Cancer J Clin.* 2005;55:10-30.
4. Damle RN, Wasil T, Fais F, et al. Ig V gene mutation status and CD38 expression as novel prognostic indicators in chronic lymphocytic leukemia. *Blood.* 1999;94:1840-1847.
5. Hamblin TJ, Davis Z, Gardiner A, et al. Unmutated Ig V(H) genes are associated with a more aggressive form of chronic lymphocytic leukemia. *Blood.* 1999;94:1848-1854.
6. Rassenti LZ, Huynh L, Toy TL, et al. ZAP-70 compared with immunoglobulin heavy-chain gene mutation status as a predictor of disease progression in chronic lymphocytic leukemia. *N Engl J Med.* 2004;351:893-901.
7. Juliusson G, Oscier DG, Fitchett M, et al. Prognostic subgroups in B-cell chronic lymphocytic leukemia defined by specific chromosomal abnormalities. *N Engl J Med.* 1990;323:720-724.
8. Dohner H, Stilgenbauer S, Benner A, et al. Genomic aberrations and survival in chronic lymphocytic leukemia. *N Engl J Med.* 2000;343:1910-1916.
9. Rai KR, Sawitsky A, Cronkite EP, et al. Clinical staging of chronic lymphocytic leukemia. *Blood.* 1975;46:219-234.
10. Binet JL, Auquier A, Dighiero G, et al. A new prognostic classification of chronic lymphocytic leukemia derived from a multivariate survival analysis. *Cancer.* 1981;48:198-206.
11. Ibrahim S, Keating M, Do KA, et al. CD38 expression as an important prognostic factor in B-cell chronic lymphocytic leukemia. *Blood.* 2001;98:181-186.
12. Crespo M, Bosch F, Villamor N, et al. ZAP-70 expression as a surrogate for immunoglobulin-variable-region mutations in chronic lymphocytic leukemia. *N Engl J Med.* 2003;348:1764-1775.
13. Dighiero G, Maloum K, Desablens B, et al. Chlorambucil in indolent chronic lymphocytic leukemia. French Cooperative Group on Chronic Lymphocytic Leukemia. *N Engl J Med.* 1998;338:1506-1514.

14. Rai KR, Peterson BL, Appelbaum FR, et al. Fludarabine compared with chlorambucil as primary therapy for chronic lymphocytic leukemia. *N Engl J Med.* 2000;343:1750-1757.
15. Kalil N, Cheson BD. Chronic lymphocytic leukemia. *Oncologist.* 1999;4:352-369.
16. O'Brien SM, Kantarjian H, Thomas DA, et al. Rituximab dose-escalation trial in chronic lymphocytic leukemia. *J Clin Oncol.* 2001;19:2165-2170.
17. Keating MJ, Flinn I, Jain V, et al. Therapeutic role of alemtuzumab (Campath-1H) in patients who have failed fludarabine: results of a large international study. *Blood.* 2002; 99:3554-3561.
18. O'Brien SM, Kantarjian HM, Cortes J, et al. Results of the fludarabine and cyclophosphamide combination regimen in chronic lymphocytic leukemia. *J Clin Oncol.* 2001;19:1414-1420.
19. Byrd JC, Peterson BL, Morrison VA, et al. Randomized phase 2 study of fludarabine with concurrent versus sequential treatment with rituximab in symptomatic, untreated patients with B-cell chronic lymphocytic leukemia: results from Cancer and Leukemia Group B 9712 (CALGB 9712). *Blood.* 2003;101:6-14.
20. Keating MJ, O'Brien S, Albitar M, et al. Early results of chemoimmunotherapy regimen of fludarabine, cyclophosphamide and ritoximab as initial therapy for chronic lymphocytic leukemia. *J Clin Oncol.* 2005;23:4079-4088.
21. Wierda W, O'Brien S, Wen S, et al. Chemoimmunotherapy with fludarabine, cyclophosphamide and ritoximab for relapsed and refractory chronic lymphocytic leukemia. *J Clin Oncol.* 2005;23:4070-4078.
22. Cooperative Group for the Study of Immunoglobulin in Chronic Lymphocytic Leukemia. Intravenous immunoglobulin for the prevention of infection in chronic lymphocytic leukemia. A randomized, controlled clinical trial. *N Engl J Med.* 1988;319:902-907.
23. Weiss RB, Freiman J, Kweder SL, et al. Hemolytic anemia after fludarabine therapy for chronic lymphocytic leukemia. *J Clin Oncol.* 1998;16:1885-1889.
24. Ozer H, Armitage JO, Bennett CL, et al. 2000 update of recommendations for the use of hematopoietic colony-stimulating factors: evidence-based, clinical practice guidelines. American Society of Clinical Oncology Growth Factors Expert Panel. *J Clin Oncol.* 2000;18:3558-3585.

CHAPTER 6

Myeloproliferative Disorders

Introduction

- The most recent WHO classification describes seven myeloproliferative disorders:[1-8]
  - Chronic myeloid (or myelogenous) leukemia (CML)
  - Polycythemia vera
  - Essential thrombocythemia
  - Chronic idiopathic myelofibrosis (with extramedullary hematopoiesis)
  - Chronic neutrophilic leukemia
  - Chronic eosinophilic leukemia (and the hypereosinophilic syndrome)
  - Chronic myeloproliferative disease, unclassifiable
- These diseases are clonal hematopoietic stem cell disorders characterized by proliferation of one or more of the myeloid lineages (ie, granulocytic, erythroid, megakaryocytic) in the bone marrow.
- The proliferation of the myeloid lineages in the bone marrow results in increased numbers of neutrophils, red blood cells, and/or platelets in the peripheral blood.
- Common clinical features include hepatomegaly, splenomegaly, and the potential to evolve to AML.

CML

- Definition
  - A myeloproliferative disorder caused by a balanced translocation between the long arms of chromosomes 9 and 22: t(9;22)(q34;q11)
  - The shortened chromosome 22 resulting from this reciprocal translocation is called the "Philadelphia chromosome" (Figure 6-1).

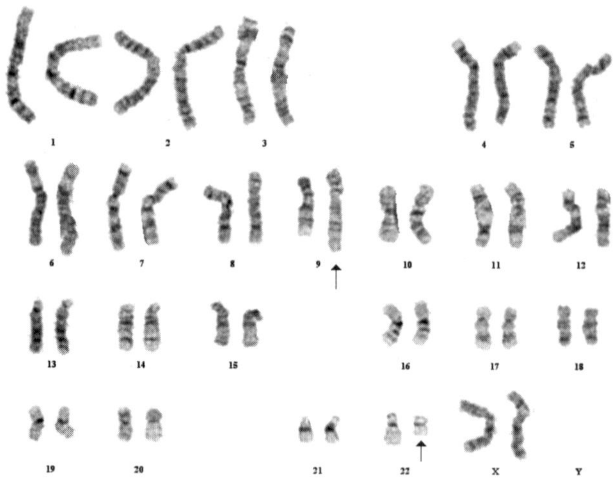

Figure 6-1: Karyotype of a patient with chronic myeloid leukemia. The arrows point to the reciprocal translocation between chromosomes 9 and 22. The shortened chromosome 22 is referred to as the Philadelphia chromosome.

- Epidemiology
  - In the United States, an estimated 4,600 new cases will occur in 2005.[9]
  - Incidence: 1.6 cases/100,000 per year[10]
  - Median age at diagnosis is 53 years.[11]
  - M:F = 1.3:1[10]
  - Risk factor: radiation exposure[10]
- Natural history
  - Three phases—a chronic phase, an accelerated phase, and a blastic phase—are typically described (Table 6-1).[2]
  - Typically, the natural history involves progression from chronic phase to accelerated phase to blastic phase. Some patients, however, may "skip" a phase (eg, go directly from chronic phase to blastic phase, or present in blastic phase).
  - Without treatment, progression from the chronic phase to the blastic phase generally takes about 3–5 years.

Table 6-1: World Health Organization Diagnostic Criteria of the Three Phases of Chronic Myeloid Leukemia

Chronic phase—not meeting criteria for accelerated or blastic phase
Accelerated phase—any of the following: • Blasts 10–19% of white blood cells in peripheral blood and/or of nucleated bone marrow cells • Peripheral blood basophils ≥20% • Persistent thrombocytopenia (<100,000/μL) unrelated to therapy, or persistent thrombocytosis (>1,000,000/μL) unresponsive to therapy • Increasing spleen size and increasing white blood cell count unresponsive to therapy • Cytogenetic evidence of clonal evolution (defined in text) • Megakaryocytic proliferation that occurs in sizeable sheets and clusters, marked reticulin or collagen fibrosis, and severe granulocytic dysplasia should be considered as suggestive of accelerated phase. However, these findings have not yet been analyzed in large studies to determine whether they are independent criteria for accelerated phase because they often occur in association with the other features listed.
Blastic phase—any of the following: • Blasts ≥20% of peripheral blood white blood cells or nucleated bone marrow cells • Extramedullary blast proliferation • Large foci or clusters of blasts in the bone marrow biopsy

Modified with permission from Jaffe et al. *Pathology and Genetics of Tumours of Haematopoietic and Lymphoid Tissues.* Lyon: IARC Press; 2001.

- About two thirds of patients progress to myeloid blast crisis, whereas the other one third have lymphoid blast crisis.

- Genetics and pathophysiology
  - The Philadelphia chromosome (Ph)
    - The *BCR* (breakpoint cluster region) gene from chromosome 22 is translocated next to the *ABL* gene from chromosome 9. This fusion gene results in the expression of BCR-ABL mRNA, which is translated to a functional BCR-ABL protein. This protein is a constitutive tyrosine kinase.[12,13]

- Different breakpoints exist in the *BCR* gene and result in production of either a 190-kd BCR-ABL fusion protein or a 210-kd BCR-ABL fusion protein (Figure 6-2). These two fusion proteins can be distinguished using PCR methods. In patients with CML, the p210 variant is nearly always present.[12,13]
- The BCR-ABL protein acts through a number of molecular pathways to give the mutant clone a survival advantage over normal hematopoietic cells.[11]

• Clonal evolution
- The leukemic clone has the tendency to acquire other genetic mutations in addition to the Ph chromosome.
- The term "clonal evolution" refers to the occurrence of other genetic mutations in addition to the Ph chromosome during the evolution to blast crisis.
- These mutations are detected in 5–10% of patients who otherwise meet criteria for chronic phase dis-

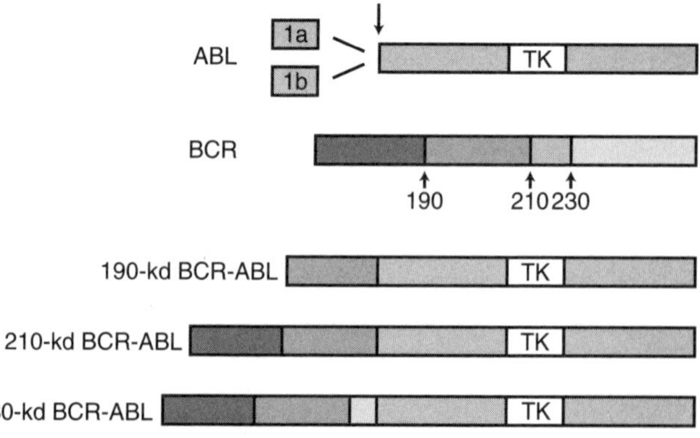

Figure 6-2: Structure of BCR-ABL fusion proteins. The structure of the wild-type ABL and BCR proteins is shown, with the site of the breakpoints in each marked by the arrows. The sizes of the fusion proteins differ depending on the amount of the BCR sequence that is retained. The length of the ABL sequence is the same in all cases. ABL has two alternative first exons (1a and 1b). TK denotes the tyrosine kinase domain. Reprinted with permission from Sawyers CL. Chronic myeloid leukemia. *N Engl J Med.* 1999;340:1330-1340.

ease, in 30% of patients who meet criteria for accelerated phase disease, and in 50–80% of patients who meet criteria for blastic phase disease.[14]

- Although any additional mutation is generally described as clonal evolution, the following are some of the commonly described mutations:[10,14]
    - Duplication of Ph chromosome
    - t(3;21)
    - Monosomy 7
    - Trisomy 8
    - Isochromosome 17 (causes a deletion of tumor suppressor gene *p53*)
    - Trisomy 19
    - Trisomy 20
    - Deletion of 20q (20q−)
    - Mutations or deletions of tumor suppressor gene *p16*

- Clinical features
    - Symptoms
        - Many patients are asymptomatic, and the diagnosis is made when a CBC performed for other reasons shows leukocytosis.
        - Constitutional symptoms such as fatigue, weight loss, and night sweats may occur.
        - High leukocyte counts rarely may lead to thrombotic complications and priapism.
    - Signs: splenomegaly is common
    - Laboratory findings
        - Leukocytosis, with WBC counts often in the range of 150,000–200,000/μL, is common.
            - Most of the leukocytes are neutrophils or their precursors, such as promyelocytes, myelocytes, metamyelocytes, and bands (Figure 6-3).
            - Eosinophils and basophils are also commonly increased in number.
        - In the chronic phase, the platelet count is usually normal or increased. In the blastic phase, thrombocytopenia may occur.

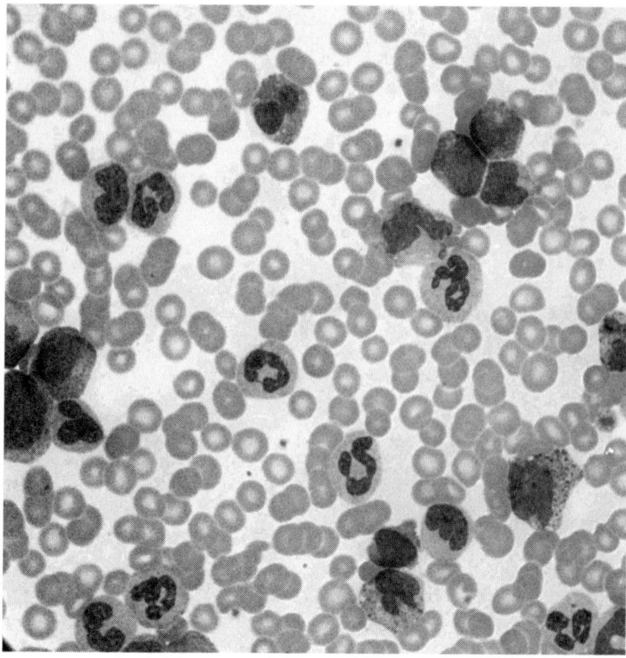

Figure 6-3: Peripheral smear of a patient with chronic myeloid leukemia. Leukocytosis is present. The white cells are neutrophils, bands, metamyelocytes, myelocytes, and promyelocytes. An eosinophil and a basophil are also present.

    - Mild anemia is common in the chronic phase.
    - Neutrophils have decreased leukocyte alkaline phosphatase.
- Pathology[2]
  - Morphology of bone marrow (Figure 6-4)
    - Hypercellular
    - Increased numbers of neutrophils and their precursors
    - The number of blasts depends on the phase.
    - Megakaryocytes tend to be small and to have hypolobulated nuclei.
    - Reticulin fibrosis is common.

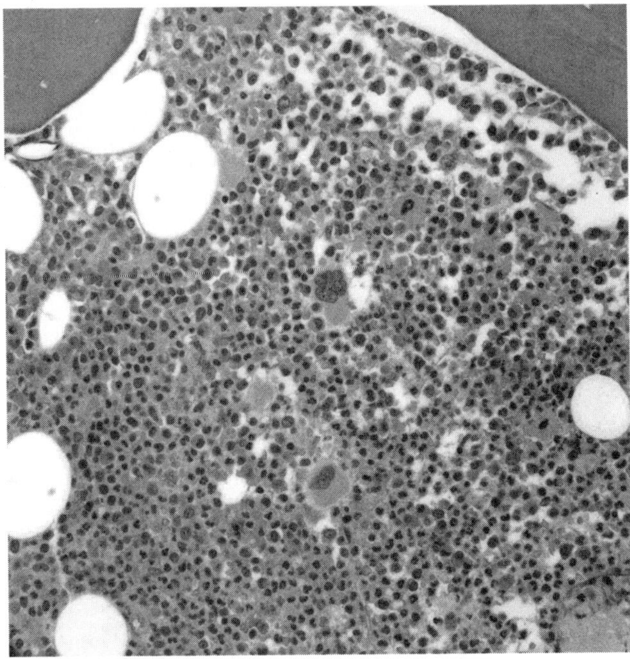

Figure 6-4: Bone marrow biopsy in a patient with chronic myeloid leukemia. The biopsy specimen is hypercellular with increased neutrophils and their precursors. Hypolobulated, small megakaryocytes are also present.

    - "Sea-blue histiocytes," which tend to stand out on low-power views, are characteristic.
  - Immunophenotype: in about 70% of cases of blast crisis, the blast lineage is myeloid, whereas in the remainder it is lymphoid.
- Diagnostic evaluation
  - In a patient in whom CML is suspected clinically, usually because of elevated peripheral blood counts, the following evaluation should be performed:
    - CBC with peripheral blood smear and manual differential, blood chemistries, uric acid

    - Bone marrow aspirate and biopsy with conventional karyotyping and molecular testing for the Ph chromosome (FISH and PCR) (Figure 6-5)
- Assessment of response[15]
    - Response to therapy is measured by monitoring peripheral blood counts, the appearance of the bone marrow, and the genetic abnormalities as detected by conventional karyotyping and molecular testing such as FISH and PCR.
    - Hematologic remission: return of peripheral blood counts and bone marrow morphology to normal

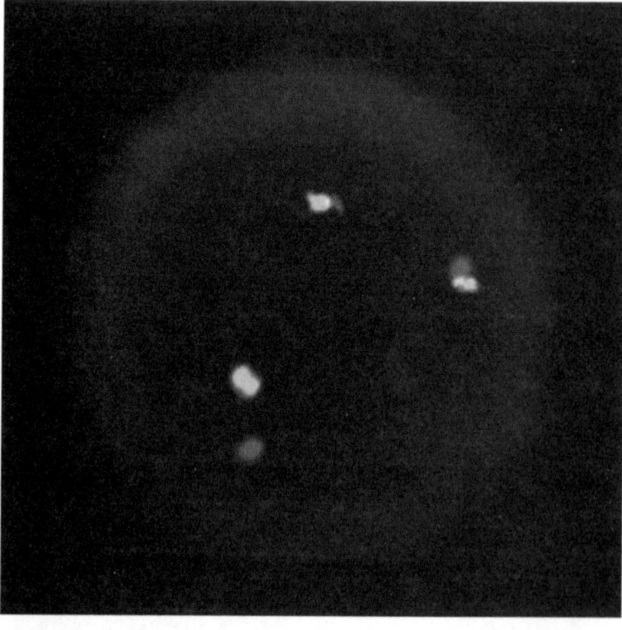

Figure 6-5: Interphase cell from a fluorescence in situ hybridization (FISH) analysis of the same patient with chronic myeloid leukemia. The DNA probe for the *ABL* gene region on chromosome 9 is directly labeled in red and the probe for the *BCR* gene region on chromosome 22 in green. The *ABL-BCR* gene fusion on the derivative 9 and the *BCR-ABL* gene fusion on the derivative 22 display red-green fusion signals.

- Cytogenetic remission: disappearance of the Ph chromosome
  - Major — 0–34% Ph-positive cells
    - Complete — 0% Ph-positive cells
    - Partial — 1–34% Ph-positive cells
  - Minor — 35–90% Ph-positive cells
- Molecular remission: disappearance of *BCR-ABL* gene as detected by PCR

- Treatment
  - Cytoreductive therapy
    - Cytoreductive therapy refers to the use of myelosuppressive drugs to decrease the circulating WBC count and thereby minimize the risk of thrombotic complications that can occur as a result of leukostasis.
    - Use of cytoreductive agents usually does not lead to cytogenetic remission (ie, the Ph chromosome persists) and does not affect the rate of progression to blastic phase.
    - Hydroxyurea and busulfan are cytoreductive agents, with hydroxyurea generally being preferred because it improved the duration of hematologic remission and median survival compared with busulfan in a randomized trial.[16]
    - The dose of hydroxyurea ranges from 250–1,500 mg PO twice daily, with doses adjusted based on peripheral blood counts.
    - Hydroxyurea is often used to lower the WBC count to below 20,000/μL before interferon alfa or imatinib mesylate is started.
    - Tumor lysis syndrome prophylaxis with allopurinol should generally be administered during therapy with hydroxyurea.
  - Interferon alfa
    - Unlike hydroxyurea and busulfan, interferon alfa can induce not only hematologic remissions but also cytogenetic remissions in patients with chronic phase CML.[16]
    - With single-agent interferon alfa therapy, the percentage of patients in whom cytogenetic remission

occurs is approximately 10–25%, and the percentage of patients alive at 5 years is approximately 50%.[16-19]

- Dose and administration
  - The target dose of interferon alfa is 5 million U/m^2 SC daily.
  - Often, lower doses are used initially until tolerance to side effects occurs.
  - Higher doses result in higher rates of cytogenetic response.
  - The WBC count should be maintained at between 2,000 and 5,000/μL.
  - Acetaminophen and antidepressants may be useful to minimize fevers and depression, respectively.
- Side effects: fevers, flu-like symptoms, fatigue, weight loss, depression. The flu-like symptoms often improve after several weeks of therapy.

- Interferon alfa plus cytarabine
  - In two trials—one in France and the other in Italy—patients with chronic phase CML were randomized to receive interferon alfa alone or with SC cytarabine. In the French trial, the addition of cytarabine improved the rates of hematologic remission, cytogenetic remission, and 3-year survival.[17] However, in the Italian trial, the addition of cytarabine improved the rate of major cytogenetic remission but not 5-year survival.[19]
  - In a large randomized trial, the combination of interferon alfa plus cytarabine was found to be inferior to therapy with imatinib mesylate.[20]
- Imatinib mesylate (Gleevec®)
  - Mechanism
    - Binds to three tyrosine kinases—*BCR-ABL*, the receptor for platelet-derived growth factor (PDGFR), and c-kit—at the adenosine triphosphate (ATP) binding site
    - Inhibits phosphorylation of proteins involved in *BCR-ABL* signal transduction

- Efficacy
  - In patients with chronic phase CML refractory to or intolerant of interferon, imatinib mesylate results in a complete hematologic response rate of greater than 95% and a major cytogenetic response rate of 60%.[15,21]
  - In patients with accelerated phase CML, imatinib mesylate results in a complete hematologic response rate of 82% and a major cytogenetic response rate of 24%.[22]
  - In patients with myeloid blastic phase CML, imatinib mesylate results in a complete hematologic response rate of 8–11% and a major cytogenetic response rate of 16%. Unfortunately, in responding patients, the median time to relapse is only about 3 months.[23,24]
  - In previously untreated patients with chronic phase CML, imatinib mesylate results in a complete hematologic response rate of 95%, a major cytogenetic response rate of 85%, and an 18-month progression-free survival rate of 97%. In a randomized trial, these results were superior to those seen with the combination of interferon alfa and cytarabine.[20]
  - Based on these data, imatinib mesylate has become the standard initial therapy for patients with CML.
- Dose and administration
  - For patients in chronic phase, the recommended initial dose is 400 mg PO daily. Dose adjustments must be made for cytopenias or other toxicities.
  - For patients in accelerated or blast phase, the recommended initial dose is 600 mg PO daily.
  - Before imatinib mesylate is initiated, hydroxyurea is often administered to lower the WBC count to below 20,000/μL.
  - The use of higher doses of imatinib mesylate in chronic phase CML is being investigated.

  - Side effects: myelosuppression and cytopenias, edema, skin rash, nausea/vomiting, elevated liver function tests, and others
- Allogeneic HCT
  - High-dose chemotherapy, with or without total body irradiation, followed by allogeneic HCT is the only known curative therapy for patients with CML.
  - Only 15–20% of patients with CML are candidates for allogeneic HCT from HLA-matched related donors because of age limitations and the low probability of having an HLA-matched sibling donor. An additional 10–15% of patients can receive bone marrow from an unrelated donor identified by bone marrow donor registries.[11]
  - Factors affecting outcome after transplantation
    - Phase of CML: patients who undergo transplantation during chronic phase have a higher likelihood of survival than do those who undergo transplantation during the accelerated phase or blast crisis.[25]
    - Duration of disease: patients who undergo transplantation within 1 year of diagnosis have a higher likelihood of survival than do those who undergo transplantation later.[25,26]
    - Patient age: younger patients have better outcomes than older patients.[27,28]
    - Because it may be advantageous to perform allogeneic HCT within the first year after diagnosis, HLA typing should be performed in all patients younger than 55 years of age and their siblings soon after the diagnosis of CML is made.
    - In patients younger than 55 years of age with an HLA-matched sibling donor, the optimal therapy is not known. Allogeneic HCT may cure about two thirds of patients but is associated with a mortality rate of about 10–20% within the first 100 days. Treatment with imatinib mesylate is less toxic but may not cure the disease.

- Graft-versus-leukemia effect: transplanted hematopoietic cells have antileukemic activity and contribute to maintaining remissions
  - When transplantations are performed with bone marrow depleted of T lymphocytes, the incidence of graft-versus-host disease declines, but the CML relapses more frequently.[29]
  - Donor lymphocyte infusions can induce CRs in patients who experience relapse after allogeneic HCT.[30]
- Conclusions
  - Before the development of imatinib mesylate, the only therapeutic options for controlling CML and modifying the rate of progression to blast crisis were interferon alfa and allogeneic HCT.
  - Imatinib mesylate is superior to interferon alfa and should generally be considered first-line therapy.
  - In young patients with HLA-matched donors, the decision about whether to continue imatinib mesylate or to proceed to allogeneic HCT is difficult for patients and their physicians. Longer follow-up in patients treated with imatinib mesylate will help guide patients and physicians in making this decision.

Polycythemia Vera

- Definition: a myeloproliferative disorder that arises in a clonal hematopoietic stem cell and is characterized by excessive red cell production[5]
- Epidemiology[5]
  - Incidence: 8–10 new cases per million population per year
  - Mean age at diagnosis is 60 years.
- Pathophysiology
  - Erythroid progenitor cells acquire the ability to proliferate in the absence of erythropoietin.
  - The red cell mass increases, resulting in hyperviscosity, which in turn causes thrombosis.

- Clinical features[5,10]
  - Symptoms
    - Venous or arterial thromboses (eg, extremity thrombosis; mesenteric, portal, or splenic vein thrombosis; myocardial infarction; stroke)
    - Neurologic symptoms: headaches, dizziness, visual disturbances, paresthesias (erythromelalgia)
    - Pruritus (classically induced by a warm bath)
    - Bleeding: epistaxis, gastrointestinal bleeds
    - Gout
  - Signs: plethora (70%), splenomegaly (70%), hepatomegaly (40%), hypertension, cutaneous ulcers
  - Laboratory
    - Elevated hemoglobin and hematocrit. The WBC count and platelet count are also commonly elevated.
    - Leukocyte alkaline phosphatase score may be elevated.
    - Lactate dehydrogenase, uric acid, and vitamin B_{12} levels may be elevated.
    - The erythropoietin level is usually low (suppressed by bone marrow's independent production of erythrocytes), although it can be normal.
    - A few laboratories can test the ability of bone marrow– or blood-derived erythroid progenitors to form colonies in serum-containing cultures in the absence of erythropoietin. This is called "endogenous erythroid colony formation." This characteristic feature is a minor diagnostic criterion.
- Pathology: bone marrow examination[5]
  - There are no pathognomonic features on bone marrow examination.
  - Common findings include hypercellularity, hyperplasia of erythroid precursors and of megakaryo-cytes, abnormal megakaryocytes (large cells with hyperlobated nuclei), and reticulin fibrosis.
  - Karyotypic analysis is useful in confirming the diagnosis if a clonal mutation is detected (and useful in excluding CML). Chromosomal abnormalities,

including trisomy 8, trisomy 9, and 20q−, can be detected in 15–80% of patients and are more common as the disease progresses.

- Diagnosis
  - Differential diagnosis: Table 6-2 lists selected causes of an elevated hematocrit.
  - Diagnostic evaluation of the patient with an elevated hematocrit (Note: not all of these tests should be performed in every patient with an elevated hematocrit. Testing should be individualized based on the clinical features of the patient.)
    - Red cell mass determination
      - Nuclear medicine physicians perform this test. A small volume of the patient's red cells are incubated with chromium-51 and reinjected into the patient. Plasma volume is measured simultaneously using albumin labeled with iodine-131. The volume of distribution of the red blood cells is then determined, and the red cell mass is calculated. A red cell mass more

Table 6-2: Selected Causes of an Elevated Hematocrit

Cause
Increased red cell mass
Polycythemia vera
Secondary polycythemia
Hypoxia
Chronic lung disease
Obstructive sleep apnea
High altitude
Erythropoietin-secreting lesions
Renal tumors or cysts
Hepatocellular carcinoma
Cerebellar hemangioblastoma
Others
High-affinity hemoglobinopathy
Decreased plasma volume
Dehydration (diuretics, alcohol)
Gaisbock's syndrome (hypertension and elevated hematocrit)

than 125% of the value predicted for that individual is considered indicative of polycythemia.
        - Because a hematocrit above 60% (or hemoglobin >18.5 g/dL) in men or a hematocrit above 55% (or hemoglobin >16.5 g/dL) in women nearly always indicates true polycythemia, red cell mass determination may be unnecessary in these patients.
    - Bone marrow aspirate and biopsy with cytogenetic analysis
    - Test for endogenous erythroid colony formation in vitro
    - Serum erythropoietin level
    - Evaluation of lung function: chest radiograph, pulmonary function tests, arterial blood gas, sleep study
    - Oxygen dissociation curve (to rule out high-affinity hemoglobinopathy)
  - WHO diagnostic criteria[5] (Table 6-3)
- Course and prognosis[10]
  - Without treatment, the median survival is only 18 months, because of the high incidence of fatal thromboembolic events.
  - With phlebotomy and platelet-lowering treatments, the median survival improves significantly; patients often live for more than 10 years.
  - Risk factors for thrombosis
    - Age greater than 60 years
    - History of previous venous or arterial thrombosis
    - High rate of phlebotomy
    - High hemoglobin or platelet count in the postoperative state
  - Phases
    - Proliferative phase: splenomegaly, marrow hyperplasia, erythrocytosis, thrombocytosis
    - Fibrotic phase: bone marrow fibrosis and impaired hematopoiesis occur
    - Postpolycythemic myeloid metaplasia: progressive hepatosplenomegaly due to extramedullary hematopoiesis, advanced bone marrow fibrosis, pancytopenia

Table 6-3: WHO Diagnostic Criteria for Polycythemia Vera

Category	Criteria
Al	Elevated red blood cell mass >25% above the mean normal predicted value, or hemoglobin >18.5 g/dL in men or >16.5 g/dL in women
A2	No cause of secondary erythrocytosis, including —Absence of familial erythrocytosis —No elevation of erythropoietin due to: Hypoxia High oxygen affinity hemoglobin Truncated erythropoietin receptor Inappropriate erythropoietin production by tumor
A3	Splenomegaly
A4	Clonal genetic abnormality other than Philadelphia chromosome or *BCR-ABL* fusion gene in marrow cells
A5	Endogenous erythroid colony formation in vitro
Bl	Thrombocytosis >400,000/μL
B2	White blood cell count >12,000/μL
B3	Bone marrow biopsy showing panmyelosis with prominent erythroid and megakaryocytic proliferation
B4	Low serum erythropoietin level

Polycythemia vera is diagnosed when Al + A2 and any other category A criterion are present, or when Al + A2 and any two criteria of category B are present.

WHO, World Health Organization.

Modified with permission from Jaffe et al. *Pathology and Genetics of Tumours of Haematopoietic and Lymphoid Tissues.* Lyon: IARC Press; 2001.

- Transformation to AML occurs in 1–3.5% of patients treated with phlebotomy alone, although the use of hydroxyurea or alkylating agents may increase the rate of transformation.

- Treatment
  - Phlebotomy
    - Lowering the hemoglobin and hematocrit to the normal range decreases viscosity, thereby reducing the risk of thromboembolic complications.
    - Initially, phlebotomy may be performed weekly to achieve rapid reduction of the hemoglobin and hematocrit.
    - Once the desired hemoglobin and hematocrit are achieved, phlebotomy may be performed less frequently (eg, monthly or every other month) in order to maintain the hemoglobin and hematocrit within the desired range.
    - Repeated phlebotomies induce iron deficiency. Iron should not be replaced in these patients. The ferritin is usually kept below 50.
    - The target hematocrit in a man should be less than 45%; the target hematocrit in a woman should be less than 42%.[31]
  - Aspirin
    - High-dose aspirin (eg, 900 mg/day) may cause bleeding complications and is probably not safe in patients with polycythemia vera.[32]
    - Low-dose aspirin, on the other hand, may help prevent thromboembolic complications. In the European Collaboration on Low-Dose Aspirin in Polycythemia Vera (ECLAP) study, low-dose aspirin (100 mg daily) lowered the rate of thrombosis in patients with polycythemia vera.[33] The rate of major bleeding was not increased in the aspirin-treated patients. One criticism leveled against this study is that phlebotomy was not adequate, because 25% of patients had hematocrit levels higher than 48% during follow-up. Thus, it seems plausible that the benefit of aspirin may have been negligible if more aggressive phlebotomy had been performed.[31] As a general rule, however, based on the results of the ECLAP trial, it seems reasonable to recommend

low-dose aspirin (eg, 81–100 mg daily) to polycythemia vera patients who have no contraindications to aspirin therapy.

- Cytoreductive agents
  - Principles
    - The Polycythemia Vera Study Group found that aggressive initial phlebotomy without cytoreductive therapy and without aspirin therapy increases the risk of thrombosis, especially in those patients already at high risk for thrombosis.
    - Therefore, in high-risk patients, particularly those older than 60 years of age and/or those with a personal history of thrombosis, cytoreductive therapy given simultaneously with phlebotomy is recommended.
  - Hydroxyurea
    - Effects
      - May reduce rate of thrombosis when given concurrently with phlebotomy
      - May reduce size of spleen
      - May lower the platelet count
    - Side effects
      - May increase the risk of acute leukemia
      - May cause severe cytopenias
      - May cause mucocutaneous ulcers
  - Interferon alfa, busulfan, and ^{32}P may also be used to control erythrocytosis but are used less commonly than hydroxyurea in the United States.[34]
  - The prostaglandin synthetase inhibitor anagrelide may be used to lower elevated platelet counts.
- Transplantation
  - Allogeneic HCT may reverse bone marrow fibrosis.
  - Small studies indicate that selected young patients with polycythemia vera may achieve long-term CRs and survival.
- Splenectomy: may be used in later stages of disease when progressive splenomegaly and cytopenias develop

- Summary
  - Several algorithms for the management of polycythemia have been proposed.[10,35-37]
  - The fact that none of these is in complete agreement with the others indicates that the optimal management of patients with polycythemia vera has yet to be defined. The considerable variation in practice patterns among hematologists in the United States also supports this conclusion.[34]
  - In general, patients with polycythemia vera should undergo phlebotomy to maintain the hematocrit at less than 45% in men and less than 42% in women. Low-dose aspirin therapy should be considered in patients who lack contraindications to aspirin. Cytoreductive therapy should be considered in patients at high risk for thrombosis (ie, those older than 60 years of age and those with a previous history of thrombosis). The choice of cytoreductive therapy should be individualized. Hydroxyurea, interferon alfa, anagrelide, busulfan, and ^{32}P are all options.

Essential Thrombocythemia

- Epidemiology[10]
  - The most common myeloproliferative disorder in the United States
  - Incidence: about 2.5 per 100,000 per year
  - Median age at diagnosis is 60 years.
- WHO diagnostic criteria[7] (Table 6-4)
- Pathophysiology
  - High platelet counts may cause microvascular occlusion, resulting in thromboses.
  - High platelet counts also may cause depletion of large von Willebrand factor multimers in the plasma, resulting in hemorrhage.
- Clinical features[10]
  - Symptoms
    - Many patients are asymptomatic, and the diagnosis is suggested by an elevated platelet count detected incidentally.

Table 6-4: WHO Diagnostic Criteria for Essential Thrombocythemia

Positive criteria

1. Sustained platelet count ≥600,000/μL
2. Bone marrow biopsy specimen showing proliferation mainly of the megakaryocytic lineage, with increased numbers of enlarged, mature megakaryocytes

Exclusion criteria

1. No evidence of polycythemia vera: normal red cell mass or hemoglobin <18.5 g/dL in men or <16.5 g/dL in women
2. No evidence of iron deficiency: stainable iron in marrow, normal serum ferritin, or normal mean corpuscular volume
3. No evidence of chronic myeloid leukemia: cytogenetics and fluorescent *in situ* hybridization or polymerase chain reaction indicate absence of Philadelphia chromosome and *BCR-ABL* fusion gene
4. No evidence of chronic idiopathic myelofibrosis: minimal reticulin fibrosis and no collagen fibrosis
5. No evidence of myelodysplastic syndrome: no del(5q), t(3;3)(q21;q26), and inv(3)(q21;q26), no granulocytic dysplasia, and few micromegakaryocytes
6. No evidence of reactive thrombocytosis (eg, from underlying infection, inflammation, neoplasm, or prior splenectomy)

WHO, World Health Organization.

Modified with permission from Jaffe et al. *Pathology and Genetics of Tumours of Haematopoietic and Lymphoid Tissues.* Lyon: IARC Press; 2001.

- Thrombosis
  - Arterial (eg, stroke, myocardial infarction, spontaneous abortion)
  - Venous (eg, extremity thrombosis, hepatic or portal vein thrombosis)
- Hemorrhage (eg, epistaxis, gastrointestinal hemorrhage)
- Vasomotor (eg, central nervous system disturbances [headaches, dizziness, cognitive deficits, seizures], burning dysesthesia of the palms and soles [erythromelalgia], cutaneous ulcers)

- Signs: splenomegaly and hepatomegaly may occur

- Laboratory
  - Leukocyte alkaline phosphatase score usually elevated
    - Mild leukocytosis may occur.
    - Peripheral blood smear may show giant platelets.
    - Bone marrow usually shows hypercellularity, with increased numbers of large megakaryocytes with hyperlobulated nuclei. The karyotype is normal in 95% of cases.
- Natural history
  - During the first decade after diagnosis, between 10% and 50% of patients experience a thrombotic episode, and 4% experience a hemorrhagic complication.[10]
  - As in polycythemia vera, risk factors for thrombotic complications include age greater than 60 years and a history of thromboembolism.[38,39]
  - About 10% of patients transform to a different myeloproliferative disorder. For example, patients may develop erythrocytosis and an elevated red cell mass as occurs in polycythemia vera. Alternatively, patients may develop bone marrow fibrosis and myeloid metaplasia as in chronic idiopathic myelofibrosis.[40]
  - In a small minority of cases, the disease will transform to AML. This risk of transformation to AML may be increased by the use of hydroxyurea,[41] although whether hydroxyurea truly increases the risk of transformation is debatable.[42]

- Treatment
  - Principles
    - Drug therapy to lower the platelet count is not absolutely necessary in all patients. Asymptomatic patients younger than 60 years of age with no history of thrombosis and platelet counts under 1.5 million/μL may have a risk of thrombosis similar to that of age-matched controls.[43] For this reason, it is reasonable to consider withholding cytoreductive

therapy in low-risk patients, particularly if other cardiovascular risk factors (eg, hypertension, hypercholesterolemia, diabetes, smoking) are absent.[37]

- Low-dose aspirin may be considered in an attempt to reduce the risk of thrombosis. However, unlike in polycythemia vera, no controlled trials have demonstrated a benefit from the use of aspirin in patients with essential thrombocythemia. Furthermore, aspirin may increase the risk of bleeding.
- Thrombotic and hemorrhagic events should generally be managed as they are managed in patients without essential thrombocythemia (eg, heparin, aspirin, thrombolytic agents as indicated).
- In patients with markedly elevated platelet counts, consideration may be given to emergent plateletpheresis.
- In patients with poorly controlled hemorrhage, consideration may be given to platelet transfusions and desmopressin (DDAVP), cryoprecipitate, or factor VIII concentrate for acquired von Willebrand disease.

- Platelet-lowering drugs
  - Hydroxyurea
    - Efficacy: in a randomized trial of 114 high-risk (age >60 years or history of thrombosis) patients with essential thrombocythemia, use of hydroxyurea to keep platelet counts below 600,000/μL significantly decreased the risk of thrombosis compared with no therapy.[44]
    - As noted above, hydroxyurea may slightly increase the rate of transformation to AML.
    - Because it is the only platelet-lowering drug proven to decrease the risk of thrombosis in high-risk patients, hydroxyurea is generally considered the drug of choice in patients who require cytoreductive therapy. However, because of its potential to increase the risk of leukemia, hydroxyurea should be used with caution in younger patients.

- Anagrelide
  - Efficacy
    - Controls the platelet count in 80–90% of patients with essential thrombocythemia
    - To date, there is no evidence that anagrelide is leukemogenic.
  - Problems
    - No controlled trials have demonstrated a decrease in the risk of thrombosis with anagrelide therapy.
    - In a retrospective series of 35 patients younger than 48 years of age treated with anagrelide, 20% suffered thrombotic complications, and 20% suffered hemorrhagic complications. In all patients who experienced a thrombotic or hemorrhagic complication, the platelet count was above 400,000/μL.[45] Thus, until more data become available, complete normalization of the platelet count should be the goal when anagrelide therapy is used.
    - Side effects include anemia, headaches, palpitations or forceful heart beats, arrhythmias, and congestive heart failure, so caution must be used in patients with underlying cardiac disease.
    - Anagrelide is not safe in pregnancy.
    - Anagrelide is more expensive than hydroxyurea.
  - Hydroxyurea versus anagrelide
    - In a recently reported trial from the United Kingdom, 809 high-risk patients with essential thrombocythemia were randomized to therapy with hydroxyurea plus low-dose aspirin or anagrelide plus low-dose aspirin. Patients treated with hydroxyurea had a lower risk of arterial thrombosis, major hemorrhage, and progression to myelofibrosis, but a higher risk of venous thrombosis. The rate of transformation to AML and overall survival

were similar, although the median follow-up of 39 months is too short to permit definitive conclusions about these end points. Hydroxyurea was better tolerated.[46]

- Given the results of the trial from the United Kingdom and other considerations, hydroxyurea is generally preferred in patients older than 60 years of age. In younger patients, in whom the leukemogenic potential of hydroxyurea is more of a concern, anagrelide may be considered.

- Interferon alfa: useful in women with essential thrombocythemia who wish to get pregnant.

Chronic Idiopathic Myelofibrosis (with Extramedullary Hematopoiesis)

- Definition: a clonal myeloproliferative disorder characterized by reactive bone marrow fibrosis, extramedullary hematopoiesis, and proliferation of one or more of the myeloid lineages (erythroid, granulocytic, and megakaryocytic) in the bone marrow[6]
- Alternative names
  - Myelofibrosis with myeloid metaplasia
  - Agnogenic myeloid metaplasia
  - Idiopathic myelofibrosis
- Pathophysiology
  - The clonal myeloproliferation is accompanied by reactive myelofibrosis and by extramedullary hematopoiesis in the spleen and other organs.
  - The reactive stromal proliferation in the bone marrow is caused by cytokines produced by the clonal myeloid cells.
  - The term "extramedullary hematopoiesis" refers to the production of blood cells in organs other than the bone marrow. The most common locations where extramedullary hematopoiesis occurs are the liver and spleen. The term "myeloid metaplasia" is used interchangeably with the term "extramedullary hematopoiesis."

- Clinical features
  - Symptoms
    - Patients are often asymptomatic.
    - Constitutional symptoms: fatigue, weight loss, night sweats, low-grade fevers, and bleeding may occur
  - Signs: marked splenomegaly is characteristic. This is usually due to extramedullary hematopoiesis, but portal hypertension may contribute.
  - Course and prognosis
    - Course is generally divided into two stages:
      - Prefibrotic stage (also known as cellular phase)
        - About 25% of patients are diagnosed in this stage.
        - Characterized by no or mild hepatomegaly and splenomegaly, mild anemia, leukocytosis, and thrombocytosis. Bone marrow shows hypercellularity, with proliferation of granulocytic and megakaryocytic precursors, but only minimal fibrosis.
      - Fibrotic stage
        - About 75% of patients are diagnosed in this stage.
        - Characterized by marked hepatomegaly and splenomegaly, marked anemia, and variable leukocyte and platelet counts. Blood smear shows prominent leukoerythroblastosis. Bone marrow shows hypocellularity, with marked collagen or reticulin fibrosis.
    - In approximately 20% of patients, the disease transforms to AML within 10 years of the onset of disease.
    - The median survival is about 3–5 years from the time of diagnosis.
    - Adverse prognostic factors[47-50]
      - Age greater than 60–70 years
      - Hgb less than 10 g/dL
      - WBC count less than 4000/μL or greater than 30,000/μL

  - Platelets less than 100,000/μL
  - Circulating blasts greater than 2%
  - Constitutional symptoms (fever, sweats, weight loss)
  - Abnormal cytogenetics
  - Increased bone marrow angiogenesis
  - Increased numbers of circulating CD34+ cells
- Pathology[6]
  - Morphology
    - Peripheral blood smear shows "leukoerythroblastosis" (teardrop-shaped erythrocytes and early red cell precursors, left-shifted granulocytic series, and giant platelets).
    - Bone marrow biopsy generally shows marked reticulin fibrosis (Figure 6-6). Megakaryocytes are large and characterized by asynchronous nuclear-cytoplasmic maturation.
    - The spleen and liver show trilineage proliferation characteristic of extramedullary hematopoiesis. Fibrosis and cirrhosis of the liver, which can lead to portal hypertension, are common.
    - Genetics: about 60% of patients have detectable cytogenetic abnormalities, including del(13q), del(20q), partial trisomy 1q, trisomy 8, and trisomy 9
- Diagnosis: at least two groups have proposed diagnostic criteria[51,52]
- Treatment
  - Principles
    - The only potentially curative therapy is allogeneic HCT.
    - Drug therapy is largely palliative and may not affect the natural history of the disease.
    - There is no "standard" drug therapy for this disease.
  - Drug therapy[37]
    - Androgens (danazol) may be used in patients with anemia or thrombocytopenia, although only the minority of patients respond.

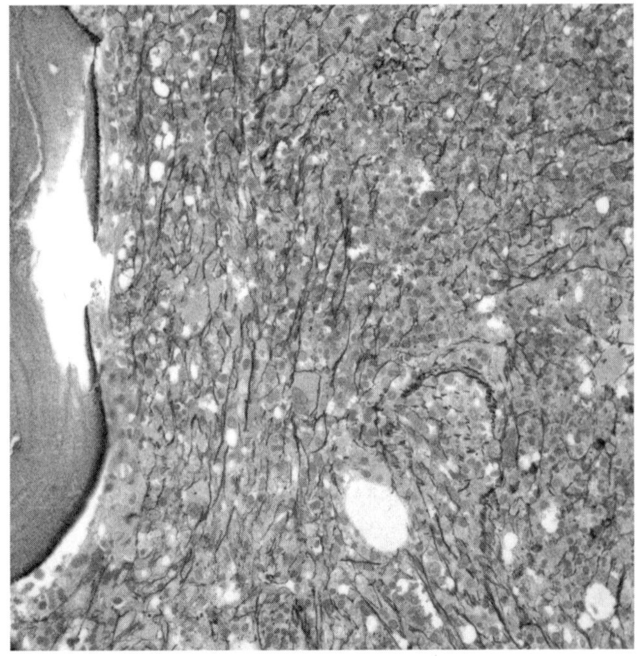

Figure 6-6: Reticulin stain on a bone marrow biopsy specimen from a patient with chronic idiopathic myelofibrosis. The marrow is hypercellular and contains increased megakaryocytes and reticulin fibrosis.

- Recombinant erythropoietin may be used for anemia.
- Corticosteroids may be used to treat constitutional symptoms.
- Hydroxyurea, interferon alfa, and other cytoreductive drugs may be used to control counts in patients with leukocytosis and thrombocytosis, and may also be helpful in reducing splenomegaly.
- Thalidomide
  - Single-agent thalidomide improves anemia, thrombocytopenia, and splenomegaly in the minority of patients.[53]

  - In a smaller phase II trial, thalidomide in combination with prednisone improved anemia and thrombocytopenia in the majority of patients, although splenomegaly improved in only a minority of patients.[54]
- Imatinib mesylate and other agents are being actively investigated.

- Splenectomy
  - May be used as palliation for symptomatic splenomegaly and hypersplenism causing anemia, although less effective for hypersplenism causing thrombocytopenia
  - Rates of morbidity (bleeding, thrombosis, infection) and mortality are relatively high, so this should be performed with caution.
- Splenic irradiation
  - May be used as palliation for symptomatic splenomegaly in patients who are poor candidates for splenectomy
  - Effective in the majority of patients, although it may be complicated by prolonged cytopenias
- Allogeneic HCT
  - Allogeneic HCT is a potentially curative therapy in patients with chronic idiopathic myelofibrosis or in patients in the myelofibrotic stages of polycythemia vera or essential thrombocythemia.
  - In a series of 56 patients undergoing allogeneic HCT in Seattle from either a related or an unrelated donor, 36 patients (56%) were alive at a median follow-up of 2.8 years. Interestingly, the prognosis for survival was not affected by whether the donor was related or unrelated.[55]
  - Nonmyeloablative transplantation is also being investigated.
- Summary
  - Patients younger than 55–60 years of age with an HLA-matched donor should be referred to a transplant center for consideration of allogeneic HCT.

- In other patients, treatment options include observation, supportive care with transfusions and growth factors, drug therapy to palliate complications of abnormal blood counts and splenomegaly, splenectomy, and splenic irradiation.

Others

- Chronic myelomonocytic leukemia
  - Definition: a clonal stem cell disorder characterized by persistent peripheral blood monocytosis (>1000/μL). Other causes of monocytosis must be excluded.[56]
  - Clinical features
    - May include hepatomegaly, splenomegaly, and leukocytosis
    - Transformation to AML occurs in about 25% of patients.
  - Treatment
    - There is no curative therapy.
    - Hydroxyurea may be used if needed to control elevated peripheral blood counts.
- Hypereosinophilic syndrome
  - Epidemiology
    - Rare
    - M:F = 9:1
    - Peak incidence in fourth decade
  - Pathophysiology
    - In some cases, the eosinophils are clonal. In such cases, proliferation of eosinophils occurs independently of stimulation by growth factors such as interleukin-3, interleukin-5, and GM-CSF.[57]
    - In other cases, the eosinophils are not clonal but instead are dependent upon stimulation by growth factors produced by other cells, such as lymphoma cells.[57]
    - Abnormalities of chromosome 4q12, resulting in fusion of the *FIP1L1* gene to the *PDGFRA* gene, have been described.[58] This fusion gene results in

the production of a constitutively activated tyrosine kinase that can transform hematopoietic cells.

- Clinical features
  - Absolute eosinophilia occurs in the peripheral blood (≥1,500 eosinophils/µL) and bone marrow.
    - The WBC count is usually less than 25,000/µL.
    - Eosinophils usually account for 30–70% of WBCs.
  - Eosinophils can infiltrate multiple organs, including the heart, lungs, spleen, skin, and nervous system, causing problems such as restrictive cardiomyopathy and interstitial lung disease.
- Treatment
  - Glucocorticoids and hydroxyurea: historically, these drugs have been used in an attempt to control the eosinophil counts and decrease symptoms.
  - Imatinib mesylate: has resulted in clinical responses in the majority of patients in a series of small trials[58-61]
  - Mepolizumab
    - An anti–interleukin-5 antibody
    - Not commercially available in the United States
    - Resulted in dramatic clinical responses in a series of three patients[62]

References

1. Vardiman JW, Brunning RD, Harris NL. Chronic myeloproliferative diseases: introduction. In: Jaffe ES, Harris NL, Stein H, Vardiman JW, eds. *Pathology and Genetics of Tumours of Haematopoietic and Lymphoid Tissues*. Lyon: IARC Press; 2001:17-19.
2. Vardiman JW, Pierre R, Thiele J, et al. Chronic myelogenous leukaemia. In: Jaffe ES, Harris NL, Stein H, Vardiman JW, eds. *Pathology and Genetics of Tumours of Haematopoietic and Lymphoid Tissues*. Lyon: IARC Press; 2001:20-26.
3. Imbert M, Bain B, Pierre R, et al. Chronic neutrophilic leukemia. In: Jaffe ES, Harris NL, Stein H, Vardiman JW, eds. *Pathology and Genetics of Tumours of Haematopoietic and Lymphoid Tissues*. Lyon: IARC Press; 2001:27-28.

4. Bain B, Pierre R, Imbert M, et al. Chronic eosinophilic leukaemia and the hypereosinophilic syndrome. In: Jaffe ES, Harris NL, Stein H, Vardiman JW, eds. *Pathology and Genetics of Tumours of Haematopoietic and Lymphoid Tissues*. Lyon: IARC Press; 2001:29-31.
5. Pierre R, Imbert M, Thiele J, et al. Polycythaemia vera. In: Jaffe ES, Harris NL, Stein H, Vardiman JW, eds. *Pathology and Genetics of Tumours of Haematopoietic and Lymphoid Tissues*. Lyon: IARC Press; 2001:32-34.
6. Thiele J, Pierre R, Imbert M, et al. Chronic idiopathic myelofibrosis. In: Jaffe ES, Harris NL, Stein H, Vardiman JW, eds. *Pathology and Genetics of Tumours of Haematopoietic and Lymphoid Tissues*. Lyon: IARC Press; 2001: 35-38.
7. Imbert M, Pierre R, Thiele J, et al. Essential thrombocythaemia. In: Jaffe ES, Harris NL, Stein H, Vardiman JW, eds. *Pathology and Genetics of Tumours of Haematopoietic and Lymphoid Tissues*. Lyon: IARC Press; 2001:39-41.
8. Thiele J, Imbert M, Pierre R, et al. Chronic myeloproliferative disease, unclassifiable. In: Jaffe ES, Harris NL, Stein H, Vardiman JW, eds. *Pathology and Genetics of Tumours of Haematopoietic and Lymphoid Tissues*. Lyon: IARC Press; 2001:42-44.
9. Jemal A, Tiwari RC, Murray T, et al. Cancer statistics, 2005. *CA Cancer J Clin*. 2005;54:8-29.
10. Linenberger M. Myeloproliferative disorders. In: George JN, Williams ME, eds. *ASH-SAP American Society of Hematology Self-Assessment Program*. Malden, MA: Blackwell Publishing; 2003:129-164.
11. Sawyers CL. Chronic myeloid leukemia. *N Engl J Med*. 1999;340:1330-1340.
12. Faderl S, Kantarjian HM, Talpaz M, Estrov Z. Clinical significance of cytogenetic abnormalities in adult acute lymphoblastic leukemia. *Blood*. 1998;91:3995-4019.
13. Radich JP. Philadelphia chromosome-positive acute lymphocytic leukemia. *Hematol Oncol Clin North Am*. 2001;15: 21-36.
14. Cortes JE, Talpaz M, Giles F, et al. Prognostic significance of cytogenetic clonal evolution in patients with chronic myelogenous leukemia on imatinib mesylate therapy. *Blood*. 2003;101:3794-3800.

15. Kantarjian H, Sawyers C, Hochhaus A, et al. Hematologic and cytogenetic responses to imatinib mesylate in chronic myelogenous leukemia. *N Engl J Med.* 2002;346:645-652.
16. Hehlmann R, Heimpel H, Hasford J, et al. Randomized comparison of interferon-alpha with busulfan and hydroxyurea in chronic myelogenous leukemia. The German CML Study Group. *Blood.* 1994;84:4064-4077.
17. Guilhot F, Chastang C, Michallet M, et al. Interferon alfa-2b combined with cytarabine versus interferon alone in chronic myelogenous leukemia. French Chronic Myeloid Leukemia Study Group. *N Engl J Med.* 1997;337:223-229.
18. Chronic Myeloid Leukemia Trialists' Collaborative Group. Interferon alfa versus chemotherapy for chronic myeloid leukemia: a meta-analysis of seven randomized trials. *J Natl Cancer Inst.* 1997;89:1616-1620.
19. Baccarani M, Rosti G, de Vivo A, et al. A randomized study of interferon-alpha versus interferon-alpha and low-dose arabinosyl cytosine in chronic myeloid leukemia. *Blood.* 2002;99:1527-1535.
20. O'Brien SG, Guilhot F, Larson RA, et al. Imatinib compared with interferon and low-dose cytarabine for newly diagnosed chronic-phase chronic myeloid leukemia. *N Engl J Med.* 2003;348:994-1004.
21. Druker BJ, Talpaz M, Resta DJ, et al. Efficacy and safety of a specific inhibitor of the BCR-ABL tyrosine kinase in chronic myeloid leukemia. *N Engl J Med.* 2001;344:1031-1037.
22. Talpaz M, Silver RT, Druker BJ, et al. Imatinib induces durable hematologic and cytogenetic responses in patients with accelerated phase chronic myeloid leukemia: results of a phase 2 study. *Blood.* 2002;99:1928-1937.
23. Druker BJ, Sawyers CL, Kantarjian H, et al. Activity of a specific inhibitor of the BCR-ABL tyrosine kinase in the blast crisis of chronic myeloid leukemia and acute lymphoblastic leukemia with the Philadelphia chromosome. *N Engl J Med.* 2001;344:1038-1042.
24. Sawyers CL, Hochhaus A, Feldman E, et al. Imatinib induces hematologic and cytogenetic responses in patients with chronic myelogenous leukemia in myeloid blast crisis: results of a phase II study. *Blood.* 2002;99:3530-3539.
25. Horowitz MM, Rowlings PA, Passweg JR. Allogeneic bone marrow transplantation for CML: a report from the

International Bone Marrow Transplant Registry. *Bone Marrow Transplant* 1996;17(suppl 3):S5-S6.
26. Report on state of the art in blood and marrow transplantation. The IBMTR/ABMTR summary slides with guide. *IBMTR/ABMTR Newsletter.* 2000;7:3-10.
27. Hansen JA, Gooley TA, Martin PJ, et al. Bone marrow transplants from unrelated donors for patients with chronic myeloid leukemia. *N Engl J Med.* 1998;338:962-968.
28. McGlave PB, Shu XO, Wen W, et al. Unrelated donor marrow transplantation for chronic myelogenous leukemia: 9 years' experience of the national marrow donor program. *Blood.* 2000;95:2219-2225.
29. Goldman JM, Gale RP, Horowitz MM, et al. Bone marrow transplantation for chronic myelogenous leukemia in chronic phase. Increased risk for relapse associated with T-cell depletion. *Ann Intern Med.* 1988;108:806-814.
30. Kolb HJ, Schattenberg A, Goldman JM, et al. Graft-versus-leukemia effect of donor lymphocyte transfusions in marrow grafted patients. European Group for Blood and Marrow Transplantation Working Party Chronic Leukemia. *Blood.* 1995;86:2041-2050.
31. Spivak J. Daily aspirin—only half the answer. *N Engl J Med.* 2004;350:99-101.
32. Tartaglia AP, Goldberg JD, Berk PD, Wasserman LR. Adverse effects of antiaggregating platelet therapy in the treatment of polycythemia vera. *Semin Hematol.* 1986;23:172-176.
33. Landolfi R, Marchioli R, Kutti J, et al. Efficacy and safety of low-dose aspirin in polycythemia vera. *N Engl J Med.* 2004;350:114-124.
34. Streiff MB, Smith B, Spivak JL. The diagnosis and management of polycythemia vera in the era since the Polycythemia Vera Study Group: a survey of American Society of Hematology members' practice patterns. *Blood.* 2002; 99:1144-1149.
35. Berk PD, Goldberg JD, Donovan PB, et al. Therapeutic recommendations in polycythemia vera based on Polycythemia Vera Study Group protocols. *Semin Hematol.* 1986;23:132-143.
36. Hoffman R. Polycythemia vera. In: Hoffman R, Benz EJ, Shattil SJ, Furie B, Cohen HJ, Silberstein LE, et al., eds. *Hematology: Basic Principles and Practice.* 3rd ed. New York: Churchill Livingstone; 2000:1130-1155.

37. Spivak JL, Barosi G, Tognoni G, et al. Chronic myeloproliferative disorders. *Hematology (Am Soc Hematol Educ Program)*. 2003:200-224.
38. Cortelazzo S, Viero P, Finazzi G, et al. Incidence and risk factors for thrombotic complications in a historical cohort of 100 patients with essential thrombocythemia. *J Clin Oncol.* 1990;8:556-562.
39. Besses C, Cervantes F, Pereira A, et al. Major vascular complications in essential thrombocythemia: a study of the predictive factors in a series of 148 patients. *Leukemia.* 1999;13:150-154.
40. Cervantes F, Alvarez-Larran A, Talarn C, et al. Myelofibrosis with myeloid metaplasia following essential thrombocythaemia: actuarial probability, presenting characteristics and evolution in a series of 195 patients. *Br J Haematol.* 2002;118:786-790.
41. Sterkers Y, Preudhomme C, Lai JL, et al. Acute myeloid leukemia and myelodysplastic syndromes following essential thrombocythemia treated with hydroxyurea: high proportion of cases with 17p deletion. *Blood.* 1998;91:616-622.
42. Finazzi G, Ruggeri M, Rodeghiero F, Barbui T. Efficacy and safety of long-term use of hydroxyurea in young patients with essential thrombocythemia and a high risk of thrombosis. *Blood.* 2003;101:3749.
43. Ruggeri M, Finazzi G, Tosetto A, et al. No treatment for low-risk thrombocythaemia: results from a prospective study. *Br J Haematol.* 1998;103:772-777.
44. Cortelazzo S, Finazzi G, Ruggeri M, et al. Hydroxyurea for patients with essential thrombocythemia and a high risk of thrombosis. *N Engl J Med.* 1995;332:1132-1136.
45. Storen EC, Tefferi A. Long-term use of anagrelide in young patients with essential thrombocythemia. *Blood.* 2001; 97:863-866.
46. Harrison CN, Campbell PJ, Buck G, et al. Hydroxyurea compared with anagrelide in high-risk essential thrombocythemia. *N Engl J Med.* 2005;353:33-45.
47. Dupriez B, Morel P, Demory JL, et al. Prognostic factors in agnogenic myeloid metaplasia: a report on 195 cases with a new scoring system. *Blood.* 1996;88:1013-1018.
48. Cervantes F, Barosi G, Demory JL, et al. Myelofibrosis with myeloid metaplasia in young individuals: disease characteristics, prognostic factors and identification of risk groups. *Br J Haematol.* 1998;102:684-690.

49. Mesa RA, Hanson CA, Rajkumar SV, et al. Evaluation and clinical correlations of bone marrow angiogenesis in myelofibrosis with myeloid metaplasia. *Blood.* 2000;96:3374-3380.
50. Barosi G, Viarengo G, Pecci A, et al. Diagnostic and clinical relevance of the number of circulating CD34(+) cells in myelofibrosis with myeloid metaplasia. *Blood.* 2001; 98:3249-3255.
51. Barosi G, Ambrosetti A, Finelli C, et al. The Italian Consensus Conference on Diagnostic Criteria for Myelofibrosis with Myeloid Metaplasia. *Br J Haematol.* 1999;104:730-737.
52. Thiele J, Kvasnicka HM, Diehl V, et al. Clinicopathological diagnosis and differential criteria of thrombocythemias in various myeloproliferative disorders by histopathology, histochemistry and immunostaining from bone marrow biopsies. *Leuk Lymphoma.* 1999;33:207-218.
53. Marchetti M, Barosi G, Balestri F, et al. Low-dose thalidomide ameliorates cytopenias and splenomegaly in myelofibrosis with myeloid metaplasia: a phase II trial. *J Clin Oncol.* 2004;22:424-431.
54. Mesa RA, Steensma DP, Pardanani A, et al. A phase 2 trial of combination low-dose thalidomide and prednisone for the treatment of myelofibrosis with myeloid metaplasia. *Blood.* 2003;101:2534-2541.
55. Deeg HJ, Gooley TA, Flowers ME, et al. Allogeneic hematopoietic stem cell transplantation for myelofibrosis. *Blood.* 2003;102:3912-3918.
56. Vardiman JW, Pierre R, Bain B, et al. Chronic myelomonocyctic leukemia. In: Jaffe ES, Harris NL, Stein H, Vardiman JW, eds. *Pathology and Genetics of Tumours of Haematopoietic and Lymphoid Tissues.* Lyon: IARC Press; 2001:49-52.
57. Schwartz RS. The hypereosinophilic syndrome and the biology of cancer. *N Engl J Med.* 2003;348:1199-1200.
58. Cools J, DeAngelo DJ, Gotlib J, et al. A tyrosine kinase created by fusion of the PDGFRA and FIP1L1 genes as a therapeutic target of imatinib in idiopathic hypereosinophilic syndrome. *N Engl J Med.* 2003;348:1201-1214.
59. Cortes J, Ault P, Koller C, et al. Efficacy of imatinib mesylate in the treatment of idiopathic hypereosinophilic syndrome. *Blood.* 2003;101:4714-4716.
60. Gleich GJ, Leiferman KM, Pardanani A, et al. Treatment of hypereosinophilic syndrome with imatinib mesilate. *Lancet.* 2002;359:1577-1578.

61. Pardanani A, Reeder T, Porrata LF, et al. Imatinib therapy for hypereosinophilic syndrome and other eosinophilic disorders. *Blood*. 2003;101:3391-3397.

62. Plotz SG, Simon HU, Darsow U, et al. Use of an anti-interleukin-5 antibody in the hypereosinophilic syndrome with eosinophilic dermatitis. *N Engl J Med*. 2003;349:2334-2339.

CHAPTER 7

Uncommon Leukemias

Prolymphocytic Leukemia (PLL) Can Be Divided into Two Subtypes: T-cell and B-cell

- T-cell PLL (T-PLL)
  - History: previously called T-cell chronic lymphocytic leukemia
  - Definition: an aggressive T-cell leukemia characterized by proliferation of small- to medium-sized prolymphocytes with a mature postthymic T-cell immunophenotype[1]
  - Epidemiology: a rare disease, accounting for about 30% of T-cell leukemias
  - Pathology[1]
    - Morphology
      - Peripheral blood smear
        - Small- to medium-sized lymphocytes with normal or irregular nuclei
        - Nucleolus often visible
        - Cytoplasmic protrusions or blebs common
      - Bone marrow usually involved with same cells
    - Immunophenotype
      - T-cell markers positive: CD2, CD3, CD7
      - 60% are CD4+ CD8−, 15% are CD4− CD8+, and 25% are CD4+ CD8+
    - Genetics
      - T-cell receptor γ and β chains are clonally rearranged.
      - 80% of cases have abnormalities of chromosome 14 at bands q11 and q32, although no cytogenetic abnormalities are pathognomonic.
  - Clinical features
    - Patients tend to be older.
    - Signs

- Hepatomegaly, splenomegaly, and lymphadenopathy
- Skin lesions may occur.
- Laboratory features: prominent lymphocytosis, anemia, and thrombocytopenia
- Treatment
  - Principles
    - There is no standard therapy.
    - There is no known curative therapy.
  - Options
    - Pentostatin: in one series, the response rate of patients with T-PLL treated with pentostatin was 45%.[2]
    - Alemtuzumab (Campath-1H)
      - In a phase II trial of 76 patients, most with disease that had progressed after first-line therapy, treatment with the humanized anti-CD52 antibody alemtuzumab resulted in an overall response rate of 51%.[3]
      - In a smaller phase II study of 39 previously treated patients in the United Kingdom, the overall response rate to alemtuzumab therapy was 76%.[4]
    - Case reports of other agents and chemotherapy regimens exist.[5]
    - Allogeneic HCT is investigational.
- Prognosis
  - An aggressive tumor that tends to be resistant to chemotherapy
  - Median survival is about 1 year.

- B-cell PLL
  - PLL[6]
  - Definition: a neoplastic proliferation of B-prolymphocytes in which prolymphocytes exceed 55% of the lymphoid cells in the blood. Transformed CLL and CLL with increased prolymphocytes must be excluded.
  - Epidemiology
    - Rare, 1% of lymphocytic leukemias
    - Occurs mostly in elderly patients.

- Pathology
  - Morphology: as in T-PLL, prolymphocytes are medium-sized lymphoid cells with prominent nucleoli.
  - Immunophenotype
    - B-cell antigens CD19, CD20, CD22, CD79a, and FMC7 are expressed.
    - Surface immunoglobulin M (IgM) with or without immunoglobulin D (IgD) is strongly expressed.
    - CD5 is expressed in one third of cases.
    - CD23 is usually absent.
  - Genetics
    - Cases have been reported with t(11;14)(q13;q32), the translocation that is typical of mantle cell lymphoma. It is quite possible that some cases reported as B-cell PLL with t(11;14) may actually represent cases of leukemic involvement of mantle cell lymphoma.
    - Other gene mutations have been described.
- Clinical features
  - Signs
    - Marked splenomegaly
    - No lymphadenopathy
  - Laboratory findings: rapid progression of lymphocytosis, anemia, and thrombocytopenia
- Treatment
  - There is no standard or curative therapy.
  - Options: CHOP (cyclophosphamide, doxorubicin, vincristine, prednisone) chemotherapy, nucleoside analogs (fludarabine, cladribine, pentostatin)
- Prognosis
  - Responds poorly to therapy
  - Survival is short.

Large Granular Lymphocyte (LGL) Leukemia

- T-cell
  - Definition: a disease characterized by persistent (>6 months) increase in the number of large granular

lymphocytes in the peripheral blood, usually numbering 2,000–20,000/μL.[7]

- Epidemiology
  - A rare disease
  - Median age at diagnosis is 55 years
- Pathology[7,8]
  - Morphology: lymphocytes are large with abundant cytoplasm and azurophilic granules
  - Immunophenotype: mature T-cell immunophenotype with expression of CD3, either CD4 or CD8 or both, and the T-cell receptor $\alpha\beta$ or $\gamma\delta$. CD57 is usually positive.
  - Genetics: clonality is usually determined by tests (Southern blot or PCR) demonstrating rearrangement of the T-cell receptor β chain gene or, less commonly, the T-cell receptor γ chain gene.
- Clinical features[7]
  - Cytopenias
    - Neutropenia
    - Anemia: pure red cell aplasia, aplastic anemia, autoimmune hemolytic anemia
    - Thrombocytopenia
  - Autoimmune phenomena
    - Positive tests for rheumatoid factor or antinuclear antibodies are common.
    - Associated with rheumatoid arthritis and Felty's syndrome
- Course and prognosis: usually tends to be indolent with survival measured in years
- Treatment
  - Indications: neutropenia or symptomatic anemia
  - There is no standard therapy. Methotrexate, cyclosporine, and cyclophosphamide have activity.

- Natural killer (NK)-cell (aggressive NK-cell leukemia)[9]
  - Definition: a disease with an aggressive clinical course characterized by systemic proliferation of NK cells. This disease must be distinguished from NK-cell LGL lymphocytosis, which is an indolent condition that, unlike T-cell LGL leukemia, does not cause cyto-

penias. In NK-cell LGL lymphocytosis, the immunophenotype of the cells is CD2+, surface CD3−, CD16+, CD56+, and CD57+.

- Epidemiology
  - Rare
  - More common among Asian teenagers and young adults
- Pathology
  - Morphology: as in T-cell LGL leukemia, the circulating lymphocytes are large with abundant cytoplasm and azurophilic granules.
  - Immunophenotype: positive for CD2 and CD56, and negative for CD3 and usually CD57
  - Genetics
  - T-cell receptor genes are not rearranged.
  - Associated with Epstein-Barr virus infection
- Clinical features: fever, constitutional symptoms, cytopenias, hepatosplenomegaly
- Course and prognosis: an aggressive disease, with survival usually less than 2 years, and often measured in weeks

Hairy Cell Leukemia

- Definition: a neoplasm of small B-lymphoid cells with oval nuclei, abundant cytoplasm, "hairy" projections, and a characteristic immunophenotype.[10]
- Epidemiology[10]
  - 2% of lymphoid leukemias in adults
  - M:F = 5:1
  - Median age at diagnosis is 55 years.
- Pathology[10]
  - Morphology
    - Hairy cells are small- to medium-sized lymphoid cells with an oval or indented nucleus, abundant pale blue cytoplasm, and circumferential "hairy" projections (Figure 7-1).
    - Hairy cells exhibit tartrate-resistant acid phosphatase (TRAP) activity (Figure 7-2). TRAP

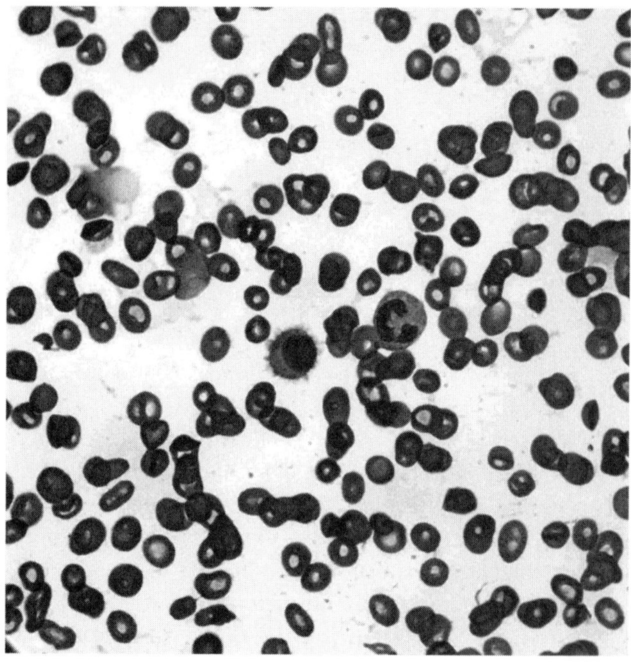

Figure 7-1: Peripheral blood smear of a patient with hairy cell leukemia. The cell in the center displays the characteristic circumferential cytoplasmic projections for which the disease is named.

activity may also occasionally be seen in other lymphoproliferative disorders.

- The bone marrow aspirate is often dry because of reticulin fibrosis. There is diffuse infiltration by lymphocytes that are spaced wider than expected, resulting in the so-called fried-egg appearance.

- Immunophenotype
  - CD11c, CD19, CD20, CD22, CD25, CD103, FMC7, and surface immunoglobulins are expressed.
  - CD5 is negative.

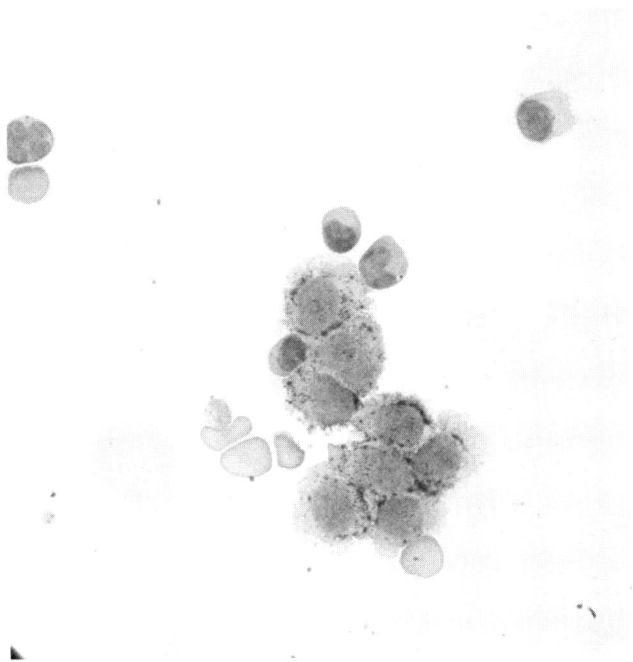

Figure 7-2: Bone marrow examination in a patient with hairy cell leukemia. The hairy cells demonstrate tartrate-resistant acid phosphatase (TRAP) activity.

- Clinical features
  - Symptoms: recurrent infections
  - Signs: splenomegaly
  - Laboratory findings: pancytopenia
- Treatment
  - Principles
    - HCL is an indolent, chronic leukemia. Many patients can survive for years without needing therapy, although most will eventually require treatment.
    - Current therapies are effective but may not be curative.
    - Indications for treatment

    - Recurrent or serious infections
    - Cytopenias: recommended thresholds of absolute neutrophils, hemoglobin, and platelet counts vary
    - Symptomatic splenomegaly
    - Constitutional symptoms
  - In patients without any of these indications, watchful waiting is a reasonable approach.
- Cladribine (2-chlorodeoxyadenosine, or 2-CdA)
  - Mechanism: a nucleoside (adenosine deaminase) analog
  - Efficacy: results in at least partial remissions in nearly all patients, and in CRs in approximately 80% of patients.[11-15] In one study with a follow-up of at least 7 years, the median duration of first response was 98 months, and the relapse rate was 36%.[15]
  - Dose: the conventional dose is 0.09–0.1 mg/kg given by IV CI over 24 hours daily for 7 days. Usually only one course of therapy is necessary. Alternative schedules have been reported.[16]
  - Toxicities: neutropenia, CD4 lymphocytopenia, fever, infections
- Pentostatin (2'-deoxycoformycin, or dCF)
  - Mechanism: an inhibitor of adenosine deaminase
  - Efficacy: like cladribine, produces CRs in approximately 80% of patients.[17-19]
  - Dose: 4 mg/m^2 IV every 2 weeks. Continue for 3–6 months until maximal bone marrow response, then two more doses given.
  - Side effects: fever, nausea/vomiting, photosensitivity, keratoconjunctivitis, infections
- Interferon alfa
  - Efficacy: interferon alfa is inferior to pentostatin in that interferon alfa produces CRs in only 11% of patients.[17] However, in patients who receive interferon alfa first and then receive pentostatin later, survival is not compromised.[19]
  - Dose

        - Interferon alfa-2a (Roferon®-A): 3 million U SC daily for 16–24 weeks, followed by 3 million U SC three times weekly
        - Interferon alfa-2b (Intron®-A): 2 million U/m^2 SC three times weekly for 6 months. Responding patients may benefit from longer durations of therapy.
    - Side effects: flu-like symptoms (fever, myalgias), depression, liver function abnormalities, possible increased risk of secondary malignancies
- Rituximab (Rituxan®): in small studies, therapy with rituximab has resulted in response rates of 25–80%.[20-22] Thus, rituximab has some activity, although its role in the treatment of hairy cell leukemia remains to be defined.
- Splenectomy: used to be the standard therapy until the mid-1980s, but not usually needed now.
- Summary
    - Cladribine and pentostatin are generally considered the best first-line agents for the treatment of hairy cell leukemia. No randomized trials have compared these two agents. Because the treatment duration with cladribine is shorter, cladribine is probably used more commonly.
    - Patients with disease progression after cladribine can still achieve remissions with pentostatin, and vice versa.
    - In general, interferon alfa is used as second- or third-line therapy after therapy with cladribine, pentostatin, or both. In patients with severe cytopenias, in whom the risk of infections complicating cladribine or pentostatin therapy may be too high, interferon alfa may be used as first-line therapy.
    - Patients with disease refractory to one nucleoside analog will often be treated with the other nucleoside analog, followed by interferon alfa, followed by splenectomy. Treatment of these patients with refractory disease is often difficult.

Adult T-cell Leukemia/Lymphoma (ATLL)

- Definition: a peripheral T-cell neoplasm caused by the retrovirus human T-cell leukemia virus type 1 (HTLV-1)[23]
- Epidemiology[23]
  - Endemic in southwestern Japan, the Caribbean, central Africa, and Central and South America
  - About 2.5% of HTLV-1 carriers in Japan develop the disease.
  - Sporadic infections occur in the United States and Europe.
  - Median age of onset in endemic areas is about 50 years.
  - M:F = 1.5:1
  - HTLV-1 is primarily transmitted from mother to child, especially through breast-feeding. Less commonly it is transmitted by sexual contact or blood transfusion.
  - The latency between initial infection with HTLV-1 and the onset of disease ranges from 20 to 60 years.
- Pathology[23]
  - Morphology
    - Malignant lymphocytes are medium-sized or large. Nucleoli are often prominent. Nuclei may be polylobulated and look like flower petals, creating so-called flower cells. These are best observed on the peripheral blood smear (Figure 7-3).
    - The bone marrow findings may range from normal to diffuse infiltration.
  - Immunophenotype
    - CD2, CD3, CD4, CD5, CD25 (strong), and HLA-DR are usually expressed. Expression of CD25 helps to distinguish ATLL from other T-cell disorders, which are usually CD25-negative.
    - CD7, CD8, and CD38 are usually negative.
  - Genetics
    - T cells have clonal rearrangements of the T-cell receptor β locus.
    - T cells show clonal integration of HTLV-1 provirus.
    - Cytogenetic abnormalities may occur and are associated with a worse prognosis.[24]

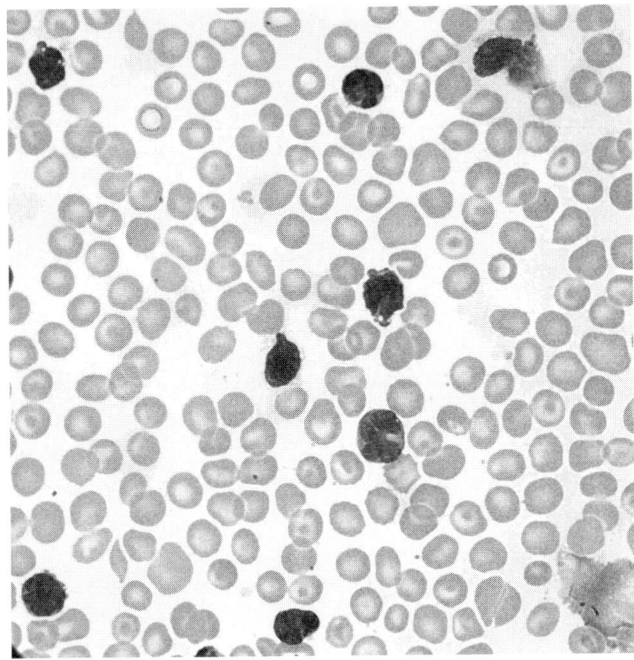

Figure 7-3: Peripheral blood smear of a patient with adult T-cell leukemia. The malignant lymphocytes contain polylobulated nuclei, producing the so-called flower cells.

- Clinical features
  - Multiple organ systems may be involved.
    - Constitutional symptoms: fever, fatigue, malaise
    - Hematologic system: lymphadenopathy, hepatomegaly, splenomegaly, marked leukocytosis and flower cells on peripheral smear, opportunistic infections due to T-cell immunodeficiency
    - Pulmonary system: pulmonary infiltrates due to infection or leukemic infiltration
    - Gastrointestinal system: diarrhea and malabsorption due to bowel involvement
    - Skin: rash (usually not itchy)
    - Central nervous system: leptomeningeal involvement may occur. Flower cells should be detectable

by cytology. The protein concentration in the spinal fluid is usually normal.

- Skeletal system: hypercalcemia and lytic bone lesions

- Subtypes[25]
  - Acute
    - Characterized by rapid onset of fever, weakness, and lymphocytosis with flower cells.
    - Multiple organ systems may be involved.
    - Hypercalcemia is common.
  - Lymphomatous: prominent lymphadenopathy without peripheral blood lymphocytosis
  - Chronic
    - Absolute lymphocyte count 400/μL or greater with flower cells
    - Lactate dehydrogenase (LDH) less than or equal to 2 times the upper limit of normal
    - Normal serum calcium
    - Lymph nodes, spleen, skin, and lungs may be involved.
    - No involvement of central nervous system, bone, gastrointestinal tract, and no ascites or effusions
  - Smoldering
    - Absolute lymphocyte count less than 400/μL
    - LDH less than or equal to 1.5 times normal
    - Normal serum calcium
    - Skin and lungs may be involved.
    - No involvement of lymph nodes, liver, spleen, central nervous system, bone, or gastrointestinal tract, and no ascites or effusions

- Prognosis
  - Survival by subtype[25]
    - The median survival of patients with the acute and lymphomatous subtypes is 6 and 10 months, respectively. Patients with these subtypes may survive only weeks.
    - The median survival of patients with the chronic and smoldering subtypes is 2 years or more. How-

ever, these subtypes may transform into the more aggressive subtypes.

- Adverse prognostic factors[8]
  - Poor performance status
  - Elevated LDH
  - Age greater than 40 years
  - Hypercalcemia
  - Increased tumor bulk
- Treatment
  - There is no standard chemotherapy regimen. Regimens used in more common types of non-Hodgkin's lymphoma are not as effective in ATLL.
  - In a recent trial conducted by the Japanese Clinical Oncology Group, 96 previously untreated patients with ATLL received three alternating chemotherapy regimens: VCAP (vincristine, cyclophosphamide, doxorubicin, and prednisone), AMP (doxorubicin, ranimustine [MCNU], and prednisone), and VECP (vindesine, etoposide, carboplatin, and prednisone).[26] Patients also received G-CSF support and intrathecal methotrexate. The overall response rate was 81%, median survival was 13 months, and 2-year survival rate was 31%. Toxicities were significant. These results compare favorably with those of previous trials conducted by the Japanese Clinical Oncology Group.
  - The combination of interferon alfa and zidovudine has also been reported to have activity.[27-29]
  - Two small series have found that allogeneic HCT is feasible and may result in at least several years of leukemia-free survival.[30,31]
  - Therapy targeting the interleukin-2 receptor CD25 is investigational.[32,33]

Mastocytosis

- Definition: a heterogeneous group of disorders characterized by the proliferation of mast cells and their accumulation in one or more organ systems[34,35]
- Epidemiology

- These are rare diseases.
- Cutaneous mastocytosis occurs more commonly in children.

- WHO classification of mastocytosis (Table 7-1)
- Cutaneous mastocytosis
  - The mast cell proliferation is confined to the skin. After stroking the skin lesions, a palpable wheal may form due to the release of histamine from the mast cells. This is called Darier's sign.
  - Three subtypes are described:
    - The most common subtype, called *urticaria pigmentosa*, is characterized by a maculopapular rash. Biopsy of the rash demonstrates aggregates of mast cells in the papillary and reticular dermis.
    - *Diffuse cutaneous mastocytosis* causes smooth, red skin or thickened skin instead of a maculopapular rash.
    - *Solitary mastocytoma of the skin* occurs most commonly in infants and usually presents as a small nodular lesion. Biopsy demonstrates sheets of mast cells. Spontaneous remission occurs in many cases. When spontaneous remission does not occur, excision may be curative.

Table 7-1: WHO Classification of Mastocytosis

Cutaneous mastocytosis
Urticaria pigmentosa
Diffuse cutaneous mastocytosis
Mastocytoma of skin
Systemic mastocytosis
Indolent systemic mastocytosis
Systemic mastocytosis with associated clonal, hematological non-mast-cell lineage disease
Aggressive systemic mastocytosis
Mast cell leukemia
Mast cell sarcoma
Extracutaneous mastocytoma

WHO, World Health Organization.

Modified with permission from Jaffe et al. *Pathology and Genetics of Tumours of Haematopoietic and Lymphoid Tissues.* Lyon: IARC Press; 2001.

- Prognosis: favorable for all three subtypes, as these diseases usually do not transform to clonal hematologic diseases.

- Systemic mastocytosis
  - In systemic mastocytosis, at least one extracutaneous organ is involved.
  - Subclassification: systemic mastocytosis may be divided into the subtypes listed in Table 7-1. In addition, *mast cell leukemia* is present when at least 20% of the nucleated cells in the marrow are mast cells. *Mast cell sarcoma* is present when a single mast cell tumor with a destructive growth pattern involves an organ besides the skin. An *extracutaneous mastocytoma* is a single mast cell tumor without a destructive growth pattern involving an organ besides the skin.[34,35]
  - Pathology: dense infiltrates of mast cells that stain for tryptase are seen in involved organs. Unlike normal mast cells, neoplastic mast cells may express CD2 and CD25.[34,35]
  - Genetics
    - Point mutations of the proto-oncogene c-*kit* are often detectable, most commonly Asp816Val.
    - However, the Asp816Val mutation of the c-*kit* gene in patients with mastocytosis may render mast cells insensitive to the c-*kit* inhibitor imatinib, probably because the mutation interferes with the binding of imatinib to c-*kit*.[36]
  - Clinical features[34,35,37]
    - Constitutional symptoms: fatigue, weight loss, fever, sweats, flushing, syncope, hypotension, tachycardia, respiratory symptoms, headache
    - Skin: rash, itching, urticaria, dermatographism
    - Bone: pain, fractures, sclerotic and lytic lesions
    - Hematologic: splenomegaly, lymphadenopathy, eosinophilia, bone marrow involvement, cytopenias. Up to 20% of patients with systemic mastocytosis develop an associated hematologic malignancy, most commonly a myeloid neoplasm like a myeloproliferative disorder or AML.

  - Gastrointestinal: abdominal pain, ulcers, hepatomegaly, cirrhosis
- Laboratory features: serum tryptase levels are usually elevated and may correlate with the burden of disease
- Prognosis: variable and difficult to predict. Patients with aggressive systemic mastocytosis, mast cell leukemia, and associated hematologic malignancies fare worse than those with other subtypes.
- Treatment
  - Cutaneous lesions may respond to psoralen-photochemotherapy (PUVA) and local corticosteroids.
  - Antihistamines and cromolyn are used for itching and other symptoms caused by histamine release.
  - Aspirin may be useful for flushing, tachycardia, and syncope, although the initial dose may cause an idiosyncratic vascular collapse.
  - Proton pump inhibitors and H1-antagonists may be used for gastrointestinal symptoms.
  - Low doses of corticosteroids may be useful for malabsorption and ascites.
  - Splenectomy may be considered in patients with symptomatic splenomegaly or hypersplenism.
  - Interferon alfa has been used with occasional success.[38-40]
  - Cladribine also had activity in one series.[41]
  - Imatinib mesylate has activity and may be considered, particularly in patients who lack the Asp816Val mutation of the c-*kit* gene.[42,43]
  - In patients with AML or mast cell leukemia, chemotherapy may be necessary. Allogeneic HCT may also be considered but is investigational.

References

1. Catovsky D, Ralfkiaer E, Müller-Hermelink HK. T-cell prolymphocytic leukaemia. In: Jaffe ES, Harris NL, Stein H, Vardiman JW, eds. *Pathology and Genetics of Tumours of Haematopoietic and Lymphoid Tissues*. Lyon: IARC Press; 2001:195-196.

2. Mercieca J, Matutes E, Dearden C, et al. The role of pentostatin in the treatment of T-cell malignancies: analysis of response rate in 145 patients according to disease subtype. *J Clin Oncol.* 1994;12:2588-2593.
3. Keating MJ, Cazin B, Coutre S, et al. Campath-1H treatment of T-cell prolymphocytic leukemia in patients for whom at least one prior chemotherapy regimen has failed. *J Clin Oncol.* 2002;20:205-213.
4. Dearden CE, Matutes E, Cazin B, et al. High remission rate in T-cell prolymphocytic leukemia with CAMPATH-1H. *Blood.* 2001;98:1721-1726.
5. Nakajima H, Oki M, Ando K. Unusual lymphoma manifestations: case 3. CD8+ T-cell prolymphocytic leukemia. *J Clin Oncol.* 2004;22:560-562.
6. Catovsky D, Montserrat E, Müller-Hermelink HK, Harris NL. B-cell prolymphocytic leukaemia. In: Jaffe ES, Harris NL, Stein H, Vardiman JW, eds. *Pathology and Genetics of Tumours of Haematopoietic and Lymphoid Tissues.* Lyon: IARC Press; 2001:131-132.
7. Chan WC, Catovsky D, Foucar K, Montserrat E. T-cell large granular lymphocyte leukaemia. In: Jaffe ES, Harris NL, Stein H, Vardiman JW, eds. *Pathology and Genetics of Tumours of Haematopoietic and Lymphoid Tissues.* Lyon: IARC Press; 2001:197-198.
8. Greer JP, Kinney MC, Loughran TP Jr. T cell and NK cell lymphoproliferative disorders. *Hematology (Am Soc Hematol Educ Program).* 2001:259-281.
9. Chan JKC, Wong KF, Jaffe ES, Ralfkiaer E. Aggressive NK-cell leukaemia. In: Jaffe ES, Harris NL, Stein H, Vardiman JW, eds. *Pathology and Genetics of Tumours of Haematopoietic and Lymphoid Tissues.* Lyon: IARC Press; 2001:198-200.
10. Foucar K, Catovsky D. Hairy cell leukaemia. In: Jaffe ES, Harris NL, Stein H, Vardiman JW, eds. *Pathology and Genetics of Tumours of Haematopoietic and Lymphoid Tissues.* Lyon: IARC Press; 2001:138-141.
11. Piro LD, Carrera CJ, Carson DA, Beutler E. Lasting remissions in hairy-cell leukemia induced by a single infusion of 2-chlorodeoxyadenosine. *N Engl J Med.* 1990;322:1117-1121.
12. Tallman MS, Hakimian D, Rademaker AW, et al. Relapse of hairy cell leukemia after 2-chlorodeoxyadenosine: long-term

follow-up of the Northwestern University experience. *Blood.* 1996;88:1954-1959.
13. Hoffman MA, Janson D, Rose E, Rai KR. Treatment of hairy-cell leukemia with cladribine: response, toxicity, and long-term follow-up. *J Clin Oncol.* 1997;15:1138-1142.
14. Saven A, Burian C, Koziol JA, Piro LD. Long-term follow-up of patients with hairy cell leukemia after cladribine treatment. *Blood.* 1998;92:1918-1926.
15. Goodman GR, Burian C, Koziol JA, Saven A. Extended follow-up of patients with hairy cell leukemia after treatment with cladribine. *J Clin Oncol.* 2003;21:891-896.
16. Lauria F, Bocchia M, Marotta G, et al. Weekly administration of 2-chlorodeoxyadenosine in patients with hairy-cell leukemia: a new treatment schedule effective and safer in preventing infectious complications. *Blood.* 1997;89:1838-1839.
17. Grever M, Kopecky K, Foucar MK, et al. Randomized comparison of pentostatin versus interferon alfa-2a in previously untreated patients with hairy cell leukemia: an intergroup study. *J Clin Oncol.* 1995;13:974-982.
18. Dearden CE, Matutes E, Hilditch BL, et al. Long-term follow-up of patients with hairy cell leukaemia after treatment with pentostatin or cladribine. *Br J Haematol.* 1999;106:515-519.
19. Flinn IW, Kopecky KJ, Foucar MK, et al. Long-term follow-up of remission duration, mortality, and second malignancies in hairy cell leukemia patients treated with pentostatin. *Blood.* 2000;96:2981-2986.
20. Hagberg H, Lundholm L. Rituximab, a chimaeric anti-CD20 monoclonal antibody, in the treatment of hairy cell leukaemia. *Br J Haematol.* 2001;115:609-611.
21. Thomas DA, O'Brien S, Bueso-Ramos C, et al. Rituximab in relapsed or refractory hairy cell leukemia. *Blood.* 2003; 102:3906-3911.
22. Nieva J, Bethel K, Saven A. Phase 2 study of rituximab in the treatment of cladribine-failed patients with hairy cell leukemia. *Blood.* 2003;102:810-813.
23. Kikuchi M, Jaffe ES, Ralfkiaer E. Adult T-cell leukaemia/lymphoma. In: Jaffe ES, Harris NL, Stein H, Vardiman JW, eds. *Pathology and Genetics of Tumours of Haematopoietic and Lymphoid Tissues.* Lyon: IARC Press; 2001:200-203.
24. Yamada Y, Hatta Y, Murata K, et al. Deletions of p15 and/or p16 genes as a poor-prognosis factor in adult T-cell leukemia. *J Clin Oncol.* 1997;15:1778-1785.

25. Shimoyama M. Diagnostic criteria and classification of clinical subtypes of adult T-cell leukaemia-lymphoma. A report from the Lymphoma Study Group (1984–87). *Br J Haematol.* 1991;79:428-437.
26. Yamada Y, Tomonaga M, Fukuda H, et al. A new G-CSF-supported combination chemotherapy, LSG15, for adult T-cell leukaemia-lymphoma: Japan Clinical Oncology Group Study 9303. *Br J Haematol.* 2001;113:375-382.
27. Gill PS, Harrington W Jr, Kaplan MH, et al. Treatment of adult T-cell leukemia-lymphoma with a combination of interferon alfa and zidovudine. *N Engl J Med.* 1995; 332:1744-1748.
28. Matutes E, Taylor GP, Cavenagh J, et al. Interferon alpha and zidovudine therapy in adult T-cell leukaemia lymphoma: response and outcome in 15 patients. *Br J Haematol.* 2001;113:779-784.
29. White JD, Wharfe G, Stewart DM, et al. The combination of zidovudine and interferon alpha-2B in the treatment of adult T-cell leukemia/lymphoma. *Leuk Lymphoma.* 2001; 40:287-294.
30. Utsunomiya A, Miyazaki Y, Takatsuka Y, et al. Improved outcome of adult T cell leukemia/lymphoma with allogeneic hematopoietic stem cell transplantation. *Bone Marrow Transplant.* 2001;27:15-20.
31. Kami M, Hamaki T, Miyakoshi S, et al. Allogeneic haematopoietic stem cell transplantation for the treatment of adult T-cell leukaemia/lymphoma. *Br J Haematol.* 2003;120:304-309.
32. Waldmann TA, White JD, Carrasquillo JA, et al. Radioimmunotherapy of interleukin-2R alpha-expressing adult T-cell leukemia with Yttrium-90-labeled anti-Tac. *Blood.* 1995;86:4063-4075.
33. Di Venuti G, Nawgiri R, Foss F. Denileukin diftitox and hyper-CVAD in the treatment of human T-cell lymphotropic virus 1-associated acute T-cell leukemia/lymphoma. *Clin Lymphoma.* 2003;4:176-178.
34. Valent P, Horny HP, Li CY, et al. Mastocytosis. In: Jaffe ES, Harris NL, Stein H, Vardiman JW, eds. *Pathology and Genetics of Tumours of Haematopoietic and Lymphoid Tissues.* Lyon: IARC Press; 2001:293-302.
35. Valent P, Horny HP, Escribano L, et al. Diagnostic criteria and classification of mastocytosis: a consensus proposal. *Leuk Res.* 2001;25:603-625.

36. Ma Y, Zeng S, Metcalfe DD, et al. The c-KIT mutation causing human mastocytosis is resistant to STI571 and other KIT kinase inhibitors; kinases with enzymatic site mutations show different inhibitor sensitivity profiles than wild-type kinases and those with regulatory-type mutations. *Blood.* 2002;99:1741-1744.
37. Bain BJ. Systemic mastocytosis and other mast cell neoplasms. *Br J Haematol.* 1999;106:9-17.
38. Kluin-Nelemans HC, Jansen JH, Breukelman H, et al. Response to interferon alfa-2b in a patient with systemic mastocytosis. *N Engl J Med.* 1992;326:619-623.
39. Worobec AS, Kirshenbaum AS, Schwartz LB, Metcalfe DD. Treatment of three patients with systemic mastocytosis with interferon alpha-2b. *Leuk Lymphoma.* 1996;22:501-508.
40. Butterfield JH. Response of severe systemic mastocytosis to interferon alpha. *Br J Dermatol.* 1998;138:489-495.
41. Kluin-Nelemans HC, Oldhoff JM, Van Doormaal JJ, et al. Cladribine therapy for systemic mastocytosis. *Blood.* 2003;102:4270-4276.
42. Pardanani A, Elliott M, Reeder T, et al. Imatinib for systemic mast-cell disease. *Lancet.* 2003;362:535-536.
43. Akin C, Fumo G, Yavuz AS, et al. A novel form of mastocytosis associated with a transmembrane c-kit mutation and response to imatinib. *Blood.* 2004;103:3222-3225.

CHAPTER 8

Aplastic Anemia

Definition

- Peripheral blood pancytopenia with a hypocellular bone marrow

Epidemiology[1]

- Rare, estimated 1,000 new cases per year in the United States
- More common in Asia than in Western countries
- Can occur at any age, but more common in young adults (ages 15–30 years) and in elderly patients (age >60 years)

Causes

- In the United States, most cases of aplastic anemia are idiopathic.
- In the diagnostic evaluation of a patient with aplastic anemia, the physician should consider testing for the potential causes listed in Table 8-1.

Pathology

- Peripheral blood smear
  - Leukopenia
  - Thrombocytopenia
  - Anemia: usually normocytic but can be macrocytic
- Bone marrow
  - Markedly hypocellular, with a decrease in all hematopoietic cells. The marrow space consists mainly of fat cells and stromal cells like fibroblasts (see Figure 8-1).
  - The morphology of the few hematopoietic cells that are present is usually normal. Overt dysplasia in a

Table 8-1: A Partial Listing of Causes of Aplastic Anemia

Idiopathic
Medications and toxins
Nonsteroidal anti-inflammatory drugs, chloramphenicol, antiepileptics, gold, sulfonamides, others
Radiation
Chemicals: benzene, solvents, insecticides
Chemotherapy drugs
Hematological diseases: paroxysmal nocturnal hemoglobinuria
Infections
Human immunodeficiency virus
Epstein-Barr virus
Cytomegalovirus
Parvovirus B19
Hepatitis viruses
Pregnancy
Inherited conditions
Fanconi's anemia, others

hypocellular bone marrow suggests a diagnosis of hypocellular MDS as opposed to aplastic anemia.

Pathophysiology

- Acquired aplastic anemia is most likely caused by cytotoxic T lymphocytes that destroy hematopoietic progenitor cells by secreting cytokines such as interferon γ and tumor necrosis factor α (TNF-α)[2]

Clinical features

- Symptoms
    - Anemia: fatigue, dyspnea
    - Leukopenia: infections
    - Thrombocytopenia: bleeding
- Signs: lymphadenopathy, hepatomegaly, and splenomegaly are generally not present.

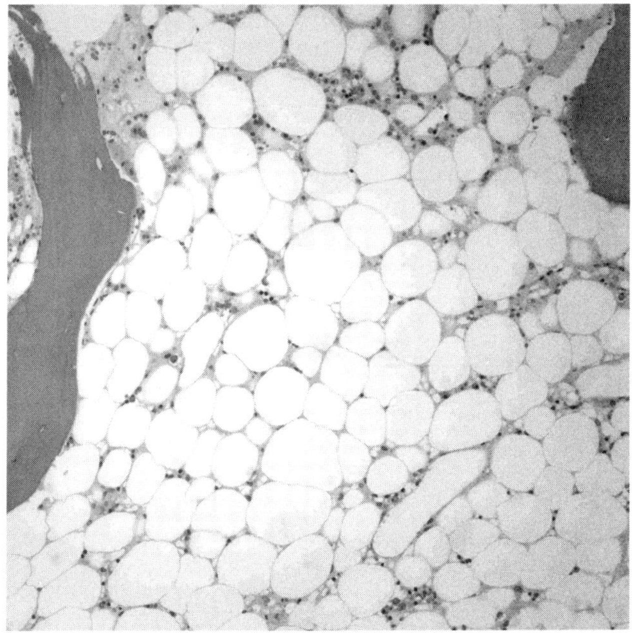

Figure 8-1: Markedly hypocellular bone marrow core biopsy specimen in a patient with aplastic anemia. The marrow consists mainly of fat cells.

Classification of the International Aplastic Anemia Study Group (Table 8-2)[1]

Diagnostic Evaluation in Patients with Pancytopenia

- *History and physical examination*: careful attention should be paid to current and recent medications, herbal supplements, history of exposure to radiation or other chemicals, recent symptoms of infection, and risk factors for human immunodeficiency virus (HIV) infection. The physical examination should include careful attention to lymphadenopathy, hepatomegaly, splenomegaly, and any musculoskeletal abnormalities.

Table 8-2: International Aplastic Anemia Study Group Classification of the Severity of Aplastic Anemia

Severity	Criteria
Moderate	Not meeting the criteria below
Severe	2 or more of the following: ANC <500/μL Platelet count <20,000/μL Reticulocyte count <20,000/μL
Super-severe	ANC <200/μL

ANC, absolute neutrophil count.

- *CBC, complete metabolic panel, reticulocyte count, and review of peripheral blood smear*: the reviewer of the peripheral blood smear should look specifically for hypersegmented neutrophils (which would suggest megaloblastic anemia), dysplastic changes (eg, hypogranular neutrophils, pelgeroid neutrophils), hairy cells, large granular lymphocytes, and leukoerythroblastosis. Any of these findings should suggest an alternate diagnosis.
- *Serum vitamin B_{12} and red cell folate levels*: to exclude their deficiencies
- Consideration of a *serologic test for HIV*
- *Bone marrow aspirate and biopsy*
  - *Flow cytometry* is useful for excluding hairy cell leukemia, LGLL, and paroxysmal nocturnal hemoglobinuria.
  - *Cytogenetic analysis*: clonal cytogenetic abnormalities may suggest myelodysplasia
- *Splenic ultrasound:* to look for splenomegaly if the physical exam is questionable (eg, in overweight patients) or suggestive of an enlarged spleen
- In patients under age 40 years, *a test for chromosome breaks* in peripheral blood lymphocytes cultured with diepoxybutane or mitomycin C should be considered to rule out Fanconi's anemia.

- *HLA-typing:* should be performed for the patient and siblings at the time of diagnosis in patients who could be considered for allogeneic HCT.

Treatment

- Immunosuppression
  - Antithymocyte globulin (ATG)
    - Mechanism
      - ATG consists of gamma globulins purified from the serum of horses, rabbits, or goats that were previously immunized with human thymocytes or thoracic duct lymphocytes.
      - ATG reduces the number of thymus-dependent lymphocytes in blood, lymph nodes, and spleen without causing severe lymphocytopenia.
      - ATG is generally administered with corticosteroids to minimize symptoms of serum sickness.
    - Forms: two forms of ATG are available in the United States—horse (equine) ATG (Atgam®, Pfizer) and rabbit ATG (Thymoglobulin®, SangStat). The US Food and Drug Administration (FDA) has approved only horse ATG for the treatment of aplastic anemia, although rabbit ATG is being actively investigated in clinical trials.
    - Efficacy
      - In the early 1980s, a randomized trial showed that ATG therapy was superior to supportive care alone.[3]
      - The response rate after ATG therapy is approximately 40–50%.[4-6]
    - Dose
      - The FDA-approved dose is 10–20 mg/kg IV daily for 8–14 days. Additional alternate-day therapy up to a total of 21 days can be administered.
      - A test dose, consisting of 0.1 mL of a 1:1,000 dilution (5 μg of horse ATG) should be given intradermally prior to the initial IV injection.

The skin test should be observed for 1 hour. A local reaction of 10 mm or more with a wheal or erythema is considered a positive test. Desensitization should be considered in patients with a positive test.
    - Other doses have been used in various clinical trials.
    - ATG is generally administered through a central venous catheter with the patient in the hospital.
  - Side effects: fever, anaphylaxis, serum sickness, others
- Cyclosporine
  - Mechanism: an inhibitor of T lymphocytes
  - Efficacy: in transfusion-dependent patients with moderate aplastic anemia, the response rate to single-agent cyclosporine is 46%.[7]
  - Side effects: renal failure, hypertension, elevated bilirubin, hemolysis, tremor, others
- Combined ATG and cyclosporine
  - Efficacy
    - The response rate with the combination of ATG and cyclosporine is approximately 70%.[4,6-9] The median time to response is about 2–3 months.[6,9] In responding patients, the risk of relapse at 2 years is about 36%.[8]
    - The percentage of patients alive 2 years after therapy is approximately 60–80%,[6,8] and the percentage of patients alive 11 years after therapy is about 55%.[6]
    - The combination of ATG and cyclosporine results in higher response rates and shorter time to response than either ATG alone[4,6] or cyclosporine alone.[7] However, overall survival is not affected because patients with disease failing single-agent therapy may respond to combination rescue therapy.
    - Patients who experience relapse after achieving remission may achieve second remissions with repeated courses of immunosuppression.
  - Doses: various dosing schedules have been reported (Table 8-3).

Table 8-3: Various Doses Used in Combination Regimens of Antithymocyte Globulin, Cyclosporine, and Corticosteroids

Trial	Horse ATG	Cyclosporine	Corticosteroid
Rosenfeld[1]	40 mg/kg IV over 4 hours daily for 4 days	6 mg/kg PO twice daily for 14 days, then adjusted to maintain level of 200–400 ng/mL until 6 months	Methylprednisolone 1 mg/kg or 40 mg (whichever was higher) daily for 10 days, then tapered over 2 weeks
Frickhofen[2]	0.75 mL/kg IV over 8–12 hours daily for 8 days	6 mg/kg PO twice daily initially. Adjusted to maintain whole-blood trough level of 500–800 ng/mL until day 28, then 200–500 ng/mL during follow-up. Continued for at least 3 months	Methylprednisolone 5 mg/kg PO or IV daily on days 1–8, then 1 mg/kg daily on days 9–14, then tapered through day 28
Marsh[3]	15 mg/kg IV daily for 5 days	5 mg/kg PO bid for at least 6 months, adjusted to maintain whole-blood trough level of 75–200 ng/mL	Prednisolone 1 mg/kg PO daily from days 5–14, then tapered over 1 week

ATG, antithymocyte globulin; IV, intravenously; PO, by mouth.

[1]Rosenfeld et al. *Blood.* 1995,85:3058-3065.

[2]Frickhofen et al. *N Engl J Med.* 1991;324:1297-1304.

[3]Marsh et al. *Blood.* 1999;93:2191-2195.

- Cyclophosphamide
  - Although preliminary reports appeared promising, in a randomized phase III trial, the combination of cyclophosphamide and cyclosporine resulted in increased morbidity and early mortality compared with the combination of ATG and cyclosporine.[10]
  - Therefore, cyclophosphamide is not considered optimal first-line therapy.
- Long-term complications of immunosuppressive therapies: patients with aplastic anemia treated with immunosuppressive drugs are at risk for the development of myelodysplasia, acute leukemia, and paroxysmal nocturnal hemoglobinuria.[8,11]

- Allogeneic HCT
  - In patients with aplastic anemia, allogeneic HCT (either bone marrow or peripheral blood stem cell) results in long-term survival rates of approximately 70%,[12] although higher rates have been reported in series from single institutions.[13,14]
  - Complications of allogeneic HCT in patients with aplastic anemia include graft rejection and graft-versus-host disease. The addition of ATG to the conditioning regimen (with cyclophosphamide) and the addition of cyclosporine to the graft-versus-host disease prophylaxis (with methotrexate) appear to reduce the risk of graft rejection.[12,13,15]
  - Most patients do not have an HLA-identical sibling donor available. Transplantation from unrelated donors has generally been less successful than transplantation from related donors, although direct comparison of the two modalities is difficult because unrelated donor transplantation has generally been performed later in the course of disease, often after failure of one or more courses of immunosuppressive therapy.[16] Thus, the role of early unrelated-donor transplantation remains to be defined. At present, unrelated-donor transplantation is generally reserved for patients with disease failing immunosuppressive therapy.
  - As age increases, outcomes after HCT worsen.

- Androgens
  - The addition of the androgen oxymetholone to ATG therapy improves response rate but does not affect overall survival.[17]
  - Androgens are not commonly used as first-line therapy.
- Supportive care
  - In cases in which a causative drug is suspected, the drug should be discontinued immediately.
  - Growth factors: filgrastim (G-CSF), sargramostim (GM-CSF), and erythropoietin may improve counts in the minority of patients, particularly in those patients with moderate (not severe) disease. However, these growth factors do not provide a cure for the disease, and their use should not delay definitive therapy in patients with severe disease.
  - Antibiotics should be started immediately in patients with neutropenia and fever.
  - Transfusions
    - The risk of graft rejection after allogeneic HCT is proportional to the number of red blood cell and platelet transfusions the patient has received prior to transplantation.[18] Therefore, in patients who are candidates for allogeneic HCT, it is prudent to use transfusions only when absolutely necessary. On the other hand, the judicious use of a few transfusions in severely anemic or bleeding patients can dramatically improve quality of life and even be life-saving without resulting in major increases in the risk of graft rejection after transplantation.
    - To minimize the risk of alloimmunization to HLAs, transfusions from relatives should be avoided.
    - Platelet transfusions may be used in patients with active bleeding or prophylactically in those with platelet counts of less than 5,000–10,000/μL.
    - Patients with aplastic anemia are at increased risk for alloimmunization, which results in refractoriness to platelet transfusions. Approaches to decrease the risk of alloimmunization to platelets include minimizing the use of platelet transfusions, using single-donor platelets rather than pooled platelets, and

leukocyte reduction of pooled platelets. In patients who become alloimmunized, as determined by failure of the platelet count to increase 1 hour after a platelet transfusion is complete, transfusion of HLA-matched platelets may be effective.
- Patients with aplastic anemia should also receive gamma-irradiated blood products to minimize the risk of transfusion-related graft-versus-host disease.
- If the patient does not have antibodies to cytomegalovirus (CMV), then CMV-negative blood products should be used.
- Granulocyte transfusions are not commonly used but may be helpful in patients with neutropenia and active infections that progress despite antibiotic therapy.

- Menstruating women with severe thrombocytopenia may be given suppressive doses of oral contraceptives to prevent excessive blood loss.

- Summary
  - The choice between immunosuppression and allogeneic HCT can be difficult for patients and their physicians. There are no randomized trials between the two treatment modalities to guide patients and their physicians. Attempts to compare the two treatment modalities retrospectively have generally favored transplantation in younger patients (ie, age <40 years), although these types of analyses are limited by their retrospective nature.[5,19,20]
  - One reasonable approach is to proceed directly to related-donor transplantation in patients younger than 40 years of age and to treat with immunosuppression in patients older than 40 years of age. In patients without a related donor, immunosuppression is usually tried first, with unrelated-donor transplantation reserved for relapse.

Prognosis

- When supportive care alone (and not immunosuppressive therapy or HCT) is used, fewer than 20% of patients survive 1 year.

- With immunosuppressive therapy, approximately 70% of patients achieve CR, although about one third eventually experience relapse and require further therapy. In one series, 55% of patients treated with immunosuppressive therapy were alive 11 years later.[6]
- Although not an option for the majority of patients, allogeneic HCT is curative in about 70% of patients.[12]
- Median survival is inversely correlated with disease severity at presentation (ie, patients with super-severe disease have the worst outcomes, followed by those with severe disease, followed by those with moderate disease).[5]

Paroxysmal Nocturnal Hemoglobinuria (PNH)

- Genetics and pathophysiology[21]
  - PNH is caused by an acquired mutation in the *PIG-A* gene, which is located on the X chromosome, in a pluripotent hematopoietic stem cell.
  - *PIG-A* encodes a protein that is essential for the synthesis of glycosylphosphatidylinositol (GPI), a lipid moiety in the plasma membrane that anchors a wide variety of proteins to the cell surface.
  - The mutation in *PIG-A* results in loss of the GPI anchor, which in turn results in loss of membrane proteins such as CD55, CD59, and others.
  - Role of CD55 and CD59
    - CD55 regulates early complement activation by inhibiting C3 convertases.
    - CD59 inhibits the assembly of the membrane attack complex C5b-C9 by interacting with C8 and C9.
    - Deficiency of CD59 on erythrocytes results in their inability to inactivate surface complement. Complement then causes intravascular hemolysis.
- Clinical features[22]
  - Intravascular hemolysis
    - Hemolytic episodes may cause fever, back pain, abdominal pain, headaches, and black urine. Surgery and infections may exacerbate hemolytic episodes.

    - Hemolysis often occurs during sleep, and the patient may awake in the mornings with black urine due to hemoglobinuria.
  - Thrombosis: venous thrombosis of an extremity, hepatic vein thrombosis (Budd-Chiari syndrome), cerebral venous sinus thrombosis, and thromboses in other locations may occur.
  - Aplastic anemia can be the initial hematologic manifestation of PNH; PNH can develop months or years after the diagnosis of aplastic anemia. Leukopenia and thrombocytopenia are often present.
  - There is likely an increased risk of acute leukemia.
  - Urinary losses may result in iron deficiency.
- Diagnosis
  - Ham's test: acidification of serum to pH 6.2 activates complement and lyses PNH cells. This test is now obsolete.
  - Flow cytometry: absence of cell-surface proteins CD55 and CD59. Many patients with bone marrow failure (perhaps 40%) have expansion of a hematopoietic PNH clone at clinical presentation.
- Course and prognosis: in one series of 80 patients, the median survival after diagnosis was 10 years, and 28% of patients survived 25 years. Fifteen percent of patients in this series experienced spontaneous clinical remissions.[23]
- Treatment
  - Treatment of hemolysis and its complications
    - High doses of corticosteroids may reduce hemolysis.
    - Iron supplementation may be needed in patients who develop iron deficiency.
    - Folate supplementation may be needed for folate deficiency from chronic hemolysis.
    - Erythropoietin therapy may be useful.
    - Red blood cell transfusions may be necessary in patients with anemia.
    - An investigational recombinant humanized monoclonal antibody called eculizumab inhibits cleavage of a terminal complement protein and de-

creases hemolysis.[21] The drug is not commercially available.

- Prophylaxis and treatment of thrombotic events
    - In patients with PNH who have never experienced a thromboembolic event, some authors have recommended prophylactic oral anticoagulation with warfarin because of the high risk of potentially fatal thrombosis.[23] However, this recommendation is not universally agreed upon.[22]
    - Patients who experience a venous thromboembolic event should be treated with heparin and warfarin. Thrombolytic therapy with tissue plasminogen activator in patients with hepatic vein thrombosis may be useful.[24]
- Treatment of bone marrow failure: immunosuppression and allogeneic HCT, as in aplastic anemia, are the treatment options for patients with bone marrow failure. Allogeneic HCT may also be considered for young patients with severe hemolysis or major thromboses.

References

1. Castro-Malaspina H, O' Reilly RJ. Aplastic anemia and myelodysplastic syndromes. In: Fauci AS, Braunwald E, Isselbacher KJ, Wilson JD, et al, eds. *Harrison's Principles of Internal Medicine*. 14th ed. New York, NY: McGraw-Hill; 1998:672-679.
2. Young NS, Maciejewski J. The pathophysiology of acquired aplastic anemia. *N Engl J Med*. 1997;336:1365-1372.
3. Champlin R, Ho W, Gale RP. Antithymocyte globulin treatment in patients with aplastic anemia: a prospective randomized trial. *N Engl J Med*. 1983;308:113-118.
4. Frickhofen N, Kaltwasser JP, Schrezenmeier H, et al. Treatment of aplastic anemia with antilymphocyte globulin and methylprednisolone with or without cyclosporine. The German Aplastic Anemia Study Group. *N Engl J Med*. 1991;324:1297-1304.
5. Paquette RL, Tebyani N, Frane M, et al. Long-term outcome of aplastic anemia in adults treated with antithymocyte globulin: comparison with bone marrow transplantation. *Blood*. 1995;85:283-290.

6. Frickhofen N, Heimpel H, Kaltwasser JP, Schrezenmeier H, German Aplastic Anemia Study Group. Antithymocyte globulin with or without cyclosporin A: 11-year follow-up of a randomized trial comparing treatments of aplastic anemia. *Blood.* 2003;101:1236-1242.
7. Marsh J, Schrezenmeier H, Marin P, et al. Prospective randomized multicenter study comparing cyclosporin alone versus the combination of antithymocyte globulin and cyclosporin for treatment of patients with nonsevere aplastic anemia: a report from the European Blood and Marrow Transplant (EBMT) Severe Aplastic Anaemia Working Party. *Blood.* 1999;93:2191-2195.
8. Rosenfeld SJ, Kimball J, Vining D, Young NS. Intensive immunosuppression with antithymocyte globulin and cyclosporine as treatment for severe acquired aplastic anemia. *Blood.* 1995;85:3058-3065.
9. Bacigalupo A, Bruno B, Saracco P, et al. Antilymphocyte globulin, cyclosporine, prednisolone, and granulocyte colony-stimulating factor for severe aplastic anemia: an update of the GITMO/EBMT study on 100 patients. European Group for Blood and Marrow Transplantation (EBMT) Working Party on Severe Aplastic Anemia and the Gruppo Italiano Trapianti di Midolio Osseo (GITMO). *Blood.* 2000;95:1931-1934.
10. Tisdale JF, Dunn DE, Geller N, et al. High-dose cyclophosphamide in severe aplastic anaemia: a randomised trial. *Lancet.* 2000;356:1554-1559.
11. Socie G, Henry-Amar M, Bacigalupo A, et al. Malignant tumors occurring after treatment of aplastic anemia. European Bone Marrow Transplantation-Severe Aplastic Anaemia Working Party. *N Engl J Med.* 1993;329:1152-1157.
12. Passweg JR, Socie G, Hinterberger W, et al. Bone marrow transplantation for severe aplastic anemia: has outcome improved? *Blood.* 1997;90:858-864.
13. Storb R, Etzioni R, Anasetti C, et al. Cyclophosphamide combined with antithymocyte globulin in preparation for allogeneic marrow transplants in patients with aplastic anemia. *Blood.* 1994;84:941-949.
14. Deeg HJ, Leisenring W, Storb R, et al. Long-term outcome after marrow transplantation for severe aplastic anemia. *Blood.* 1998;91:3637-3645.
15. Stucki A, Leisenring W, Sandmaier BM, et al. Decreased rejection and improved survival of first and second marrow

transplants for severe aplastic anemia (a 26-year retrospective analysis). *Blood.* 1998;92:2742-2749.

16. Storb RF, Lucarelli G, McSweeney PA, Childs RW. Hematopoietic cell transplantation for benign hematological disorders and solid tumors. *Hematology (Am Soc Hematol Educ Program).* 2003:372-397.
17. Bacigalupo A, Chaple M, Hows J, et al. Treatment of aplastic anaemia (AA) with antilymphocyte globulin (ALG) and methylprednisolone (MPred) with or without androgens: a randomized trial from the EBMT SAA working party. *Br J Haematol.* 1993;83:145-151.
18. Champlin RE, Horowitz MM, van Bekkum DW, et al. Graft failure following bone marrow transplantation for severe aplastic anemia: risk factors and treatment results. *Blood.* 1989;73:606-613.
19. Doney K, Leisenring W, Storb R, Appelbaum FR. Primary treatment of acquired aplastic anemia: outcomes with bone marrow transplantation and immunosuppressive therapy. Seattle Bone Marrow Transplant Team. *Ann Intern Med.* 1997;126:107-115.
20. Bacigalupo A, Brand R, Oneto R, et al. Treatment of acquired severe aplastic anemia: bone marrow transplantation compared with immunosuppressive therapy—the European Group for Blood and Marrow Transplantation experience. *Semin Hematol.* 2000;37:69-80.
21. Hillmen P, Hall C, Marsh JC, et al. Effect of eculizumab on hemolysis and transfusion requirements in patients with paroxysmal nocturnal hemoglobinuria. *N Engl J Med.* 2004;350:552-559.
22. Lottenberg R, Zumberg M. Hemolytic anemias. In: George JN, Williams ME, eds. *ASH-SAP American Society of Hematology Self-Assessment Program.* Malden, MA: Blackwell Publishing; 2003:77-115.
23. Hillmen P, Lewis SM, Bessler M, et al. Natural history of paroxysmal nocturnal hemoglobinuria. *N Engl J Med.* 1995;333:1253-1258.
24. McMullin MF, Hillmen P, Jackson J, et al. Tissue plasminogen activator for hepatic vein thrombosis in paroxysmal nocturnal haemoglobinuria. *J Intern Med.* 1994;235:85-89.

CHAPTER 9

Plasma Cell Neoplasms

WHO Classification of Plasma Cell Neoplasms (Table 9-1)[1]

Multiple Myeloma and Variants

- Definition: a malignancy of plasma cells that is generally characterized by a monoclonal protein in the serum, lytic bone lesions, hypercalcemia, and anemia
- Epidemiology
  - An estimated 15,980 new cases will occur in the United States in 2005.[2]
  - Median age at diagnosis is about 70 years.[1]
  - M = F
  - More common in blacks than in whites
- Pathology
  - Morphology[1]
    - The bone marrow contains increased numbers of plasma cells. The plasma cells may vary in appearance from normal (oval cells with blue cytoplasm, eccentric nucleus, and perinuclear clearing) to markedly abnormal (eg, with prominent nucleoli and multiple nuclei) (Figure 9-1).
    - Occasionally plasma cells may be found in the peripheral blood.
  - Immunophenotype[1]
    - Flow cytometry is generally less useful in the diagnosis of multiple myeloma than in the diagnosis and subclassification of other leukemias.
    - Malignant plasma cells typically express cytoplasmic immunoglobulin (IgG > IgA > others) but not surface immunoglobulin. CD38, CD79a, and CD138 are usually expressed.
    - CD19 and CD20 are usually negative.

Table 9-1: World Health Organization Classification of Plasma Cell Neoplasms

Plasma cell myeloma (multiple myeloma)
Variants: nonsecretory myeloma, indolent myeloma, smoldering myeloma, plasma cell leukemia
Plasmacytoma
Solitary plasmacytoma of bone
Extramedullary plasmacytoma
Monoclonal immunoglobulin deposition diseases
Primary amyloidosis
Systemic light and heavy chain deposition diseases
Light chain deposition disease
Heavy chain deposition disease
Light and heavy chain deposition disease
Osteosclerotic myeloma (POEMS syndrome)
Heavy chain diseases
Gamma heavy chain disease
Mu heavy chain disease
Alpha heavy chain disease

POEMS, polyneuropathy, organomegaly, endocrinopathy, mononoclonal gammopathy, skin changes.

Modified with permission from Jaffe et al. *Pathology and Genetics of Tumours of Haematopoietic and Lymphoid Tissues.* Lyon: IARC Press; 2001.

- Genetics[3]
  - Conventional cytogenetic analysis is often difficult in cases of multiple myeloma because of the low proliferative index of malignant plasma cells. Nevertheless, cytogenetic abnormalities can be identified in approximately 30–50% of patients.
  - FISH analysis is more sensitive than conventional karyotyping for the detection of genetic abnormalities.
  - Multiple chromosomal abnormalities have been reported, including deletions of parts or all of chromosome 13 and multiple translocations involving immunoglobulin genes.

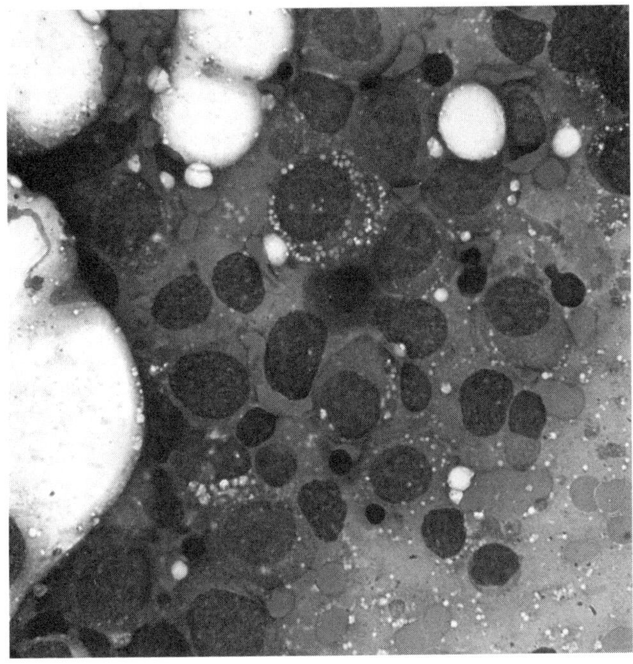

Figure 9-1: Bone marrow aspirate in a patient with multiple myeloma. Large numbers of abnormal, vacuolated plasma cells are present. Other patients with multiple myeloma will have increased numbers of normal-appearing plasma cells.

- Clinical features[4,5]
  - Common
    - Anemia: due to marrow infiltration and renal failure. The "rouleaux formation," in which the red blood cells are arranged linearly in stacks, may be seen on the peripheral blood smear (Figure 9-2).
    - Skeletal manifestations
      - Lytic bone lesions
        - Typically involve axial skeleton (skull, spine, pelvis)
        - May cause bone pain, pathologic fractures, and spinal cord compression

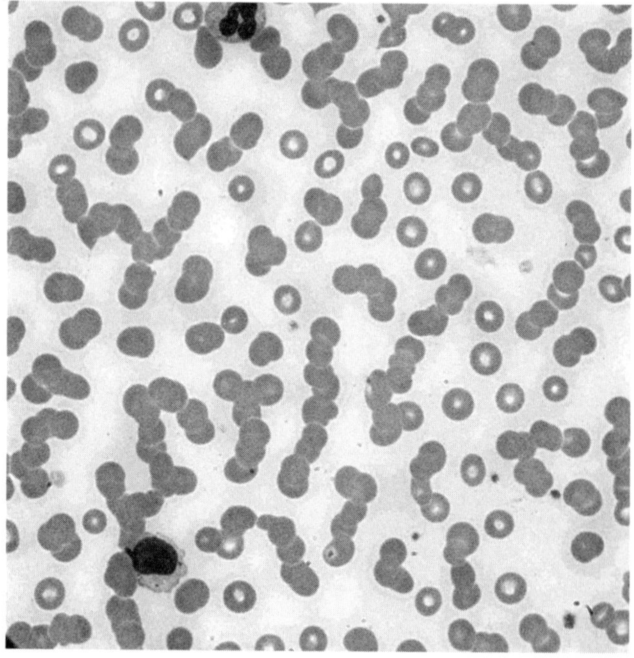

Figure 9-2: Peripheral blood smear of a patient with multiple myeloma, demonstrating the "rouleaux formation" in which the erythrocytes clump together in a linear stack.

- Because myelomatous lesions are usually purely lytic, with little blastic component, and because bone scans detect reactive bone formation, radiologic bone surveys are more effective than bone scans in detecting myeloma bone involvement.
- Osteoporosis may also occur.
- Renal failure
  - Present in about 20% of patients at diagnosis
  - Often reversible with hydration, correction of hypercalcemia, and effective chemotherapy
  - Mechanisms
    - Light chain deposition causes cast nephropathy.

    - Hypercalcemia causes nephrocalcinosis and dehydration.
    - Amyloid deposition
    - Hyperuricemia
    - Patients with multiple myeloma are at increased risk for acute renal failure caused by contrast dye used for imaging studies.
  - Recurrent bacterial infections: due to suppression of uninvolved normal immunoglobulins
  - Hypercalcemia
- Unusual
  - Hyperviscosity syndrome
  - Peripheral neuropathy
  - Bleeding: due to paraprotein interference with proteins of the coagulation cascade
- Laboratory findings: the types of monoclonal protein produced are IgG (55%), IgA (25%), immunoglobulin D (IgD) (1%), and kappa or lambda light chains only (20%). Fewer than 5% of patients have no detectable monoclonal immunoglobulin, or so-called nonsecretory myeloma.

- Diagnostic evaluation (Table 9-2)
- Diagnostic criteria[1]
  - Diagnostic criteria for multiple myeloma (Table 9-3)
  - Diagnostic criteria for monoclonal gammopathy of undetermined significance (MGUS), smoldering myeloma, and indolent myeloma (Table 9-4)
- Staging
  - The most frequently used staging system for multiple myeloma is the Durie-Salmon system (Table 9-5).[6]
  - In this system, more advanced stage correlates with increased myeloma cell mass in the body.
- Course and prognosis
  - About 20–25% of patients with MGUS eventually progress to multiple myeloma, amyloidosis, or a non-Hodgkin's lymphoma at a rate of about 1% per year.[7]
  - Many patients with smoldering myeloma live for years without evidence of progression. The median time to progression is approximately 2 years.[8]

Table 9-2: Diagnostic Evaluation of the Patient with Suspected or Newly Discovered Multiple Myeloma

- History and physical exam
- Complete blood count, complete metabolic panel, including calcium, lactate dehydrogenase, β_2-microglobulin
- Serum protein electrophoresis to identify presence or absence of monoclonal protein
- Serum immunofixation: a more sensitive test to identify presence or absence of monoclonal protein; allows identification of specific monoclonal protein involved (IgG, IgA, IgM, IgD, kappa or lambda light chains)
- 24-hour urine for protein, electrophoresis, and immunofixation
- Quantitative immunoglobulin levels in serum
- Skeletal survey
- Bone marrow aspirate and biopsy, including conventional cytogenetic analysis and fluorescent *in situ* hybridization (FISH) analysis for common molecular defects, especially deletion of chromosome 13
- ± magnetic resonance imaging (MRI) of spine

- The median survival of patients with multiple myeloma is approximately 4 years.[7]
- Prognostic factors[9,10]
  - Durie-Salmon stage: more advanced stage correlates with increased myeloma cell mass in the body
  - Cytogenetic abnormalities: monosomy 13, del(13q), and hypodiploidy are adverse prognostic factors.[11,12]
  - β_2-microglobulin: elevated values are an adverse prognostic factor. Because the kidneys excrete β_2-microglobulin, elevated levels occur in patients with renal failure; the significance of such elevated levels in the setting of renal failure is unclear.
  - Other adverse prognostic factors: advanced age, poor performance status, elevated LDH levels, elevated C-reactive protein, high plasma cell labeling index (not a widely available test), elevated soluble interleukin-6 receptor level (also not widely available), others

Table 9-3: World Health Organization Diagnostic Criteria for Multiple Myeloma

Major criteria

A. Marrow plasmacytosis >30%
B. Plasmacytoma on biopsy
C. M-component
Serum: IgG >3.5 g/dL, IgA >2 g/dL
Urine: >1 gram of Bence-Jones protein in a 24-hour urine specimen

Minor criteria

A. Marrow plasmacytosis 10–30%
B. M-component present but less than above
C. Lytic bone lesions
D. Reduced normal immunoglobulins (<50% normal)
IgG <600 mg/dL, IgA <100 mg/dL, IgM <50 mg/dL

The diagnosis of multiple myeloma requires one of the following scenarios in a symptomatic patient with progressive disease:
At least one major and one minor criterion, or
three minor criteria that must include A and B

Modified with permission from Jaffe et al. *Pathology and Genetics of Tumors of Haematopoietic and Lymphoid Tissues.* Lyon: IARC Press; 2001.

- Response criteria: historically, response criteria have varied from study to study. In 1998, new criteria were proposed to define response after HCT:[13]
  - Complete response (all of the following)
    - No evidence of monoclonal protein by serum and urine immunofixation tests, maintained for at least 6 weeks
    - Less than 5% plasma cells in bone marrow
    - No increase in size or number of lytic bone lesions
    - Disappearance of soft tissue plasmacytomas
  - Partial response (all of the following)
    - Reduction of serum and urine monoclonal protein by at least 50%, maintained for at least 6 weeks
    - Reduction of 24-hour urine light chain excretion either by 90% or greater or to less than 200 mg, maintained for at least 6 weeks

Table 9-4: World Health Organization Diagnostic Criteria for Monoclonal Gammopathy of Undetermined Significance (MGUS), Smoldering Myeloma, and Indolent Myeloma

Monoclonal gammopathy of undetermined significance (MGUS)
- Monoclonal gammopathy present
  - If monoclonal protein is IgG, level must be <3.5 g/dL
  - If monoclonal protein is IgA, level must be <2 g/dL
- Marrow plasmacytosis <10%
- No lytic bone lesions
- No myeloma-related symptoms

Smoldering myeloma: same as MGUS except:
- Monoclonal gammopathy present, and IgG >3.5 g/dL or IgA >2 g/dL
- Marrow plasmacytosis 10–30%

Indolent myeloma: same as multiple myeloma except:
- IgG <7 g/dL, IgA <5 g/dL
- No more than 3 lytic bone lesions and no compression fractures
- Normal hemoglobin, serum calcium, and creatinine
- No infections

Modified with permission from Jaffe et al. *Pathology and Genetics of Tumours of Haematopoietic and Lymphoid Tissues.* Lyon: IARC Press; 2001.

    - Reduction of soft tissue plasmacytoma, if present, by at least 50%
    - No increase in size or number of lytic bone lesions
- Treatment
  - Principles
    - There is no cure.[7]
    - The goals of therapy are to alleviate symptoms and to prolong survival.
    - For patients with MGUS, no treatment is necessary. Follow-up generally consists of checking the monoclonal protein level every 6 months to ensure stability.
    - For patients with smoldering myeloma or asymptomatic stage I multiple myeloma, delaying therapy and treating patients at the time of disease progression may not adversely affect survival.[14] A reason-

Table 9-5: Durie-Salmon Staging System for Multiple Myeloma

Stage I—all of the following: Hemoglobin >10 g/dL Serum calcium ≤12 mg/dL No lytic bone lesions, or solitary bone plasmacytoma only Low M-component production rates IgG <5 g/dL if monoclonal IgG IgA <3 g/dL if monoclonal IgA Urine light chain M component <4 g/24 hours
Stage II—not meeting criteria for stage I or III
Stage III—any of the following: Hemoglobin <8.5 g/dL Serum calcium >12 mg/dL Advanced, multiple lytic bone lesions High M-component production rates IgG >7 g/dL IgA >5 g/dL Urine light chain M-component >12 g/24 hours
Subclassification based on renal function A = serum creatinine <2 mg/dL B = serum creatinine ≥2 mg/dL

Modified with permission from Durie and Salmon. *Cancer.* 1975;36:842-854. Copyright 1975 American Cancer Society.

able approach in these patients is observation or enrollment in a clinical trial with a therapy designed to delay progression.
  - Therapy is indicated in symptomatic patients with multiple myeloma.
- Conventional chemotherapy
  - Melphalan plus prednisone
    - Efficacy[7,15,16]
      - Overall response rate 50%
      - CR rate less than 10%
      - Median survival about 2–3 years and 5-year overall survival rate about 20–25%

- Dose
  - Principles
    - There is more than one way to dose melphalan and prednisone.
    - In general, a CBC should be checked about 3 weeks after beginning melphalan. The goal is to achieve modest neutropenia at that time. Subsequent doses can be adjusted depending on the midcycle neutrophil and platelet counts.
  - Options for initial dosing
    - Melphalan 0.15 mg/kg PO daily for 7 days plus prednisone 20 mg PO three times daily for 7 days, repeat cycle every 6 weeks
    - Melphalan 0.25 mg/kg PO daily for 4 days plus prednisone 20 mg PO three times daily for 4 days, repeat cycle every 4–6 weeks
    - Melphalan 9 mg/m^2 PO daily for 4 days plus prednisone 60 mg/m^2 PO once daily for 4 days, repeat cycle every 6 weeks
  - The dose of melphalan should be reduced in patients with renal insufficiency.
- Duration: in the absence of disease progression, at least three cycles of therapy should be given. Objective responses may require more than 6 months of therapy.
- Side effects: include cytopenias and delayed engraftment in patients undergoing autologous HCT. Patients who might receive autologous HCT in the future should not be treated with melphalan.

- Combination chemotherapy
  - A variety of regimens has been developed, including infusional VAD (vincristine, doxorubicin, dexamethasone),[17] bolus VAD,[18] VBMCP (vincristine, carmustine, melphalan, cyclophosphamide, and prednisone),[15] ABCM (doxorubicin, carmustine, cyclophosphamide,

melphalan),[19] DVD (liposomal doxorubicin, vincristine, and dexamethasone),[20] and others.
- Efficacy
  - Response rates with combination chemotherapy regimens are approximately 60–70% and are superior to those achieved with melphalan and prednisone.[16]
  - However, overall survival with combination chemotherapy regimens is the same as in patients treated with melphalan and prednisone.[16]

- Thalidomide
  - Mechanism: inhibits angiogenesis
  - Efficacy
    - In patients with refractory myeloma, therapy with single-agent thalidomide results in an overall response rate of 32%.[21]
    - In patients with newly diagnosed myeloma, the combination of thalidomide and dexamethasone results in a response rate of 64–80%.[22-24]
  - Dose
    - The optimal dose of thalidomide has not been defined.
    - Most studies have used doses of approximately 200 mg PO daily. Higher doses are associated with increased toxicity.
  - Side effects: deep vein thrombosis (about 15%), peripheral neuropathy, lethargy, constipation, skin rash, bradycardia, teratogenicity, others
  - Because of the high risk of deep vein thrombosis associated with the thalidomide–dexamethasone regimen, many authors recommend prophylactic anticoagulation with warfarin.
  - At the time of this writing, the FDA has not approved thalidomide for the treatment of multiple myeloma.
- Autologous HCT
  - Efficacy

    - The median survival in patients treated with high-dose chemotherapy and autologous HCT is approximately 4–5 years.[25-27]
    - Compared with conventional chemotherapy alone, high-dose chemotherapy and autologous HCT probably improve response rates and median survival.[25,26] However, not all studies have demonstrated a survival benefit.[27]
  - Other issues
    - In order to reduce the number of myeloma cells in the blood and bone marrow, three to four cycles of chemotherapy, using a regimen that does not contain an alkylating agent, are usually administered prior to high-dose chemotherapy. The most commonly used regimen is VAD, although the thalidomide–dexamethasone combination may also be used.
    - Use of peripheral blood stem cells as opposed to bone marrow stem cells may result in more rapid engraftment and is generally preferred.
    - When used as the preparative regimen, melphalan 200 mg/m^2 is less toxic and at least as effective as the preparative regimen of melphalan 140 mg/m^2 plus 8 Gy of total body irradiation.[28]
    - In a randomized study from France, double transplantation improved survival compared with single transplantation.[17] One limitation of this study is that patients did not receive 200 mg/m^2 of melphalan as the preparative regimen.
- Allogeneic HCT
  - Potential advantages provided by allogeneic HCT are: (1) the graft is not contaminated by myeloma cells and (2) there is a graft-versus-myeloma effect.
  - Disadvantages of allogeneic HCT are its higher morbidity and mortality rates and its lack of availability to a large number of patients.
  - Nonmyeloablative transplantation theoretically should lower morbidity and mortality rates associated with intensive preparative regimens.
  - Allogeneic transplantation remains investigational in multiple myeloma.

- Bisphosphonates
  - Efficacy
    - Therapy with IV bisphosphonates such as pamidronate and zoledronic acid lowers the risk of skeletal events (pathologic fracture, spinal cord compression, and irradiation of or surgery on bone) and improves bone pain in patients with multiple myeloma.[29-31]
    - These drugs are also effective for the treatment of hypercalcemia.
  - Doses
    - Pamidronate: 90 mg IV over 2 hours every 3–4 weeks
    - Zoledronic acid: 4 mg IV over 15 minutes every 3–4 weeks
  - Side effects: nephrotoxicity (renal function should be monitored periodically), avascular necrosis of the jaw bones
- Maintenance therapy
  - In patients who respond to induction chemotherapy with VAD and do not go on to receive transplantation, maintenance therapy with prednisone 50 mg every other day improves progression-free and overall survival compared with prednisone 10 mg every other day.[32]
  - A number of trials have investigated the role of maintenance therapy with interferon alfa with conflicting results. A meta-analysis of 12 studies concluded that use of interferon alfa as maintenance therapy prolonged median time to progression by 6 months and median survival by 4 months, but that this small survival benefit came at the price of increased cost and toxicity.[33]
- Bortezomib (Velcade®)
  - Mechanism: a proteasome inhibitor
  - Efficacy
    - In patients with multiple myeloma refractory to at least two prior therapies, treatment with bortezomib results in an overall response rate of 35%.[34]

    - In patients with relapsed multiple myeloma, bortezomib improves response rates, time to progression, and overall survival compared with dexamethasone.[35]
  - Dose: 1.3 mg/m^2 IV over 3–5 seconds twice weekly for 2 weeks, followed by a 10-day rest period (days 1, 4, 8, and 11 in a 21-day cycle)
  - Side effects: fatigue, fever, nausea, vomiting, diarrhea, constipation, neutropenia, anemia, thrombocytopenia, peripheral neuropathy
  - Bortezomib has been approved by the FDA for use in patients with progression of multiple myeloma after at least one prior therapy.
- Summary
  - In patients older than 70 years of age and in those who will not be considered for autologous HCT, the combination of melphalan and prednisone is often considered the preferred therapy. In patients presenting with acute renal failure, combination chemotherapy with the VAD regimen may be preferred because reduction of melphalan dose is required.
  - In newly diagnosed patients who may be considered for autologous HCT, initial therapy usually consists of a chemotherapy regimen, such as VAD or thalidomide–dexamethasone, that does not contain an alkylating agent. Stem cells are then collected, followed by high-dose therapy with autologous HCT. In patients who do not achieve CR after the first transplant, a second transplant may be considered.
  - Most patients with multiple myeloma should be treated with either pamidronate or zoledronic acid to reduce the risk of skeletal events. These drugs have not been well studied in patients with creatinine levels above 3 mg/dL. They are not indicated in patients with MGUS, solitary plasmacytoma, or smoldering myeloma.

Plasmacytoma

- Definition: plasmacytomas are clonal proliferations of plasma cells characterized by a localized growth pattern, either within or outside of bone. If the growth is within bone, then the term "solitary plasmacytoma of bone," or "osseous plasmacytoma," is used. If the growth is outside of bone, then the term "extraosseous plasmacytoma" is used.[1]
- Clinical features
  - Symptoms: bone pain or pathologic fracture
  - Laboratory findings: some patients may have a low-level monoclonal gammopathy
  - Pathology: the lesion consists of monoclonal plasma cells
  - Treatment: radiation therapy to the affected area, followed by close observation
  - Prognosis: many patients develop multiple myeloma, especially if a monoclonal protein remains detectable after radiation therapy

Monoclonal Immunoglobulin Deposition Diseases

- Primary amyloidosis
  - Definition: a plasma cell neoplasm characterized by the presence of an abnormal immunoglobulin that forms a β-pleated sheet structure, binds Congo red with apple-green birefringence, and contains amyloid P component[1]
  - Epidemiology[1]
    - A rare disease
    - 20% of patients with amyloidosis have overt multiple myeloma.
    - 15% of patients with multiple myeloma develop amyloidosis.
  - Pathophysiology
    - Neoplastic plasma cells produce small fragments of lambda or kappa light chains. Alternatively, the neoplastic plasma cells may produce immunoglobulins that are degraded by macrophages into light chains.

- Intact monoclonal light chains and fragments of the variable regions of the light chains combine to form the fibrillary protein called amyloid.
- Amyloid is deposited in a variety of organs, resulting in organ damage and the clinical manifestations of the disease.

- Pathology[1]
  - On hematoxylin and eosin staining, amyloid is an amorphous, eosinophilic, waxy-appearing substance.
  - When stained with Congo red and viewed by polarization microscopy, the characteristic apple-green birefringence is noted.
- Clinical features[36]
  - Cardiac: cardiomegaly, congestive heart failure, conduction defects, arrhythmias, "granular sparkling" appearance on echocardiogram
  - Renal: proteinuria ranging from mild to nephrotic range, renal insufficiency
  - Gastrointestinal: hepatomegaly, splenomegaly, cholestasis, malabsorption, macroglossia
  - Skin: papules, plaques, purpura, periorbital ecchymosis
  - Neurological: peripheral neuropathy, carpal tunnel syndrome, orthostatic hypotension
  - Hematological: bleeding from factor X deficiency due to factor X binding of amyloid fibrils, monoclonal gammopathy (majority of patients)
- Diagnosis
  - The diagnosis of amyloidosis is made by the identification of amyloid in biopsy specimens of affected organs.
  - If amyloid is suspected based on clinical features, then an abdominal fat pad aspirate or a rectal biopsy may be diagnostic.
  - The bone marrow examination may reveal increased plasma cells and amyloid.
- Prognosis[36]
  - The average survival is approximately 1 year but is worse if multiple myeloma is present.

  - The major causes of death are heart disease and renal failure.
- Treatment
  - Historically, the combination of melphalan and prednisone has been used in an attempt to control amyloid deposition and preserve organ function.
  - Recent series have shown promising results with high-dose melphalan and autologous HCT.[37,38]
- Systemic light and heavy chain deposition diseases: these plasma cell neoplasms have clinical features and natural histories similar to those of primary amyloidosis. In contrast to amyloid, the immunoglobulin fragments secreted by the neoplastic plasma cells in these deposition diseases form a nonfibrillary, amorphous material that does not have a β-pleated sheet configuration, does not bind Congo red, and does not contain amyloid P component. In light chain deposition disease, kappa light chains are more frequent than lambda light chains, whereas the reverse is true in amyloidosis.

Osteosclerotic Myeloma (POEMS Syndrome)

- This rare plasma cell neoplasm is characterized by polyneuropathy (sensorimotor demyelination), organomegaly (hepatomegaly and splenomegaly), endocrinopathy (diabetes, gynecomastia, testicular atrophy, and erectile dysfunction), monoclonal gammopathy, and skin changes (hyperpigmentation, hypertrichosis). The bone marrow contains one or more "osteosclerotic plasmacytomas," which consist of clonal plasma cells adjacent to focally thickened trabecular bone and peritrabecular fibrosis. The prognosis is more favorable than in multiple myeloma.[1]

Heavy Chain Diseases[1]

- Principles
  - Heavy chain diseases are not true plasma cell neoplasms. Instead, they are variants of lymphomas.

- In these rare diseases, the malignant cells produce an incomplete, truncated heavy chain. The monoclonal protein may not be detectable by serum protein electrophoresis and may require immunofixation for detection.
- IgG (gamma heavy chain disease), IgM (mu heavy chain disease), or IgA (alpha heavy chain disease) may be produced.

- Gamma heavy chain disease
  - A variant of lymphoplasmacytic lymphoma
  - Clinical features: constitutional symptoms, autoimmune hemolytic anemia or thrombocytopenia, lymphadenopathy, splenomegaly, hepato-megaly, and peripheral eosinophilia
  - Pathology: lymph nodes contain a mix of lymphocytes, plasmacytoid lymphocytes, and plasma cells. Immunohistochemical stains demonstrate positivity for cytoplasmic gamma chain without light chains.
- Mu heavy chain disease
  - A variant of CLL
  - Clinical features: similar to CLL, although lymphadenopathy may be absent and hepatosplenomegaly more prominent
  - Pathology
    - Immunofixation shows mu chains in the serum. Urine immunofixation may show free light chains. These light chains are produced by the malignant cells but not assimilated into functional immunoglobulin molecules because of the defective mu heavy chains.
    - The bone marrow contains small, mature-appearing lymphocytes similar to those seen in CLL. In addition, characteristic vacuolated plasma cells are present.
    - The malignant cells express cytoplasmic mu heavy chains without light chains and do not express CD5.
- Alpha heavy chain disease
  - A variant of extranodal marginal zone lymphoma of mucosa-associated lymphoid tissue (MALT)

- Epidemiology: occurs primarily in areas bordering the Mediterranean Sea
- Clinical features: malabsorption and diarrhea due to involvement of the gastrointestinal tract. The disease may transform to large B-cell lymphoma.
- Pathology
  - The lamina propria of the bowel is infiltrated by plasma cells and small lymphocytes.
  - The plasma cells and marginal zone B cells express monoclonal cytoplasmic alpha chains without light chains.

References

1. Grogan TM, Van Camp B, Kyle RA, et al. Plasma cell neoplasms. In: Jaffe ES, Harris NL, Stein H, Vardiman JW, eds. *Pathology and Genetics of Tumours of Haematopoietic and Lymphoid Tissues*. Lyon: IARC Press; 2001:142-156.
2. Jemal A, Murray T, Ward E, et al. Cancer statistics, 2005. *CA Cancer J Clin*. 2005;55:10-30.
3. Dalton WS, Bergsagel PL, Kuehl WM, et al. Multiple myeloma. *Hematology (Am Soc Hematol Educ Program)*. 2001:157-177.
4. Barlogie B, Alexanian R, Jagannath S. Plasma cell dyscrasias. *JAMA*. 1992;268:2946-2951.
5. Munshi NC, Tricot G, Barlogie B. Plasma cell neoplasms. In: DeVita VT, Hellman S, Rosenberg SA, eds. *Cancer: Principles & Practice of Oncology*. 6th ed. Philadelphia, PA: Lippincott Williams & Wilkins; 2001:265-2499.
6. Durie BG, Salmon SE. A clinical staging system for multiple myeloma. Correlation of measured myeloma cell mass with presenting clinical features, response to treatment, and survival. *Cancer*. 1975;36:842-854.
7. Rajkumar SV, Kyle RA, Gertz MA. Myeloma and the newly diagnosed patient: a focus on treatment and management. *Semin Oncol*. 2002;29(suppl 17):5-10.
8. Witzig TE, Kyle RA, O'Fallon WM, Greipp PR. Detection of peripheral blood plasma cells as a predictor of disease course in patients with smouldering multiple myeloma. *Br J Haematol*. 1994;87:266-272.
9. Turesson I, Abildgaard N, Ahlgren T, et al. Prognostic evaluation in multiple myeloma: an analysis of the impact of new prognostic factors. *Br J Haematol*. 1999;106:1005-1012.

10. Desikan R, Jagannath S, Richardson P, Munshi NC. Multiple myeloma and other plasma cell dyscrasias. In: Pazdur R, Coia LR, Hoskins WJ, Wagman LD, eds. *Cancer Management: A Multidisciplinary Approach*. 8th ed. Manhasset, NY: CMP Healthcare Media; 2004:727-745.
11. Barlogie B, Jagannath S, Desikan KR, et al. Total therapy with tandem transplants for newly diagnosed multiple myeloma. *Blood*. 1999;93:55-65.
12. Facon T, Avet-Loiseau H, Guillerm G, et al. Chromosome 13 abnormalities identified by FISH analysis and serum beta2-microglobulin produce a powerful myeloma staging system for patients receiving high-dose therapy. *Blood*. 2001;97:1566-1571.
13. Blade J, Samson D, Reece D, et al. Criteria for evaluating disease response and progression in patients with multiple myeloma treated by high-dose therapy and haemopoietic stem cell transplantation. Myeloma Subcommittee of the EBMT. European Group for Blood and Marrow Transplant. *Br J Haematol*. 1998;102:1115-1123.
14. Hjorth M, Hellquist L, Holmberg E, et al. Initial versus deferred melphalan-prednisone therapy for asymptomatic multiple myeloma stage I—a randomized study. Myeloma Group of Western Sweden. *Eur J Haematol*. 1993;50:95-102.
15. Oken MM, Harrington DP, Abramson N, et al. Comparison of melphalan and prednisone with vincristine, carmustine, melphalan, cyclophosphamide, and prednisone in the treatment of multiple myeloma: results of Eastern Cooperative Oncology Group Study E2479. *Cancer*. 1997;79:1561-1567.
16. Myeloma Trialists' Collaborative Group. Combination chemotherapy versus melphalan plus prednisone as treatment for multiple myeloma: an overview of 6,633 patients from 27 randomized trials. *J Clin Oncol*. 1998;16:3832-3842.
17. Attal M, Harousseau JL, Facon T, et al. Single versus double autologous stem-cell transplantation for multiple myeloma. *N Engl J Med*. 2003;349:2495-2502.
18. Segeren CM, Sonneveld P, van der Holt B, et al. Vincristine, doxorubicin and dexamethasone (VAD) administered as rapid intravenous infusion for first-line treatment in untreated multiple myeloma. *Br J Haematol*. 1999;105:127-130.

19. MacLennan IC, Chapman C, Dunn J, Kelly K. Combined chemotherapy with ABCM versus melphalan for treatment of myelomatosis. The Medical Research Council Working Party for Leukaemia in Adults. *Lancet.* 1992;339:200-205.
20. Hussein MA, Wood L, Hsi E, et al. A phase II trial of pegylated liposomal doxorubicin, vincristine, and reduced-dose dexamethasone combination therapy in newly diagnosed multiple myeloma patients. *Cancer.* 2002;95:2160-2168.
21. Singhal S, Mehta J, Desikan R, et al. Antitumor activity of thalidomide in refractory multiple myeloma. *N Engl J Med.* 1999;341:1565-1571.
22. Rajkumar SV, Hayman S, Gertz MA, et al. Combination therapy with thalidomide plus dexamethasone for newly diagnosed myeloma. *J Clin Oncol.* 2002;20:4319-4323.
23. Weber D, Rankin K, Gavino M, et al. Thalidomide alone or with dexamethasone for previously untreated multiple myeloma. *J Clin Oncol.* 2003;21:16-19.
24. Rajkumar SV, Blood E, Vesole DH, et al. A randomised phase III trial of thalidomide plus dexamethasone versus dexamethasone in newly diagnosed multiple myeloma (E1A00): a trial coordinated by the Eastern Cooperative Oncology Group [abstract]. *J Clin Oncol.* 2004 ASCO Annual Meeting Proceedings (Post-Meeting Edition). 2004;22(July 15 supplement): 558. Abstract 6508.
25. Attal M, Harousseau JL, Stoppa AM, et al. A prospective, randomized trial of autologous bone marrow transplantation and chemotherapy in multiple myeloma. Intergroupe Francais du Myelome. *N Engl J Med.* 1996;335:91-97.
26. Child JA, Morgan GJ, Davies FE, et al. High-dose chemotherapy with hematopoietic stem-cell rescue for multiple myeloma. *N Engl J Med.* 2003;348:1875-1883.
27. Segeren CM, Sonneveld P, van der Holt B, et al. Overall and event-free survival are not improved by the use of myeloablative therapy following intensified chemotherapy in previously untreated patients with multiple myeloma: a prospective randomized phase 3 study. *Blood.* 2003;101:2144-2151.
28. Moreau P, Facon T, Attal M, et al. Comparison of 200 mg/m^2 melphalan and 8 Gy total body irradiation plus 140 mg/m^2 melphalan as conditioning regimens for peripheral blood stem cell transplantation in patients with newly diagnosed multiple myeloma: final analysis of the Intergroupe Francophone du Myelome 9502 randomized trial. *Blood.* 2002;99:731-735.

29. Berenson JR, Lichtenstein A, Porter L, et al. Efficacy of pamidronate in reducing skeletal events in patients with advanced multiple myeloma. Myeloma Aredia Study Group. *N Engl J Med.* 1996;334:488-493.
30. Berenson JR, Lichtenstein A, Porter L, et al. Long-term pamidronate treatment of advanced multiple myeloma patients reduces skeletal events. Myeloma Aredia Study Group. *J Clin Oncol.* 1998;16:593-602.
31. Rosen LS, Gordon D, Kaminski M, et al. Zoledronic acid versus pamidronate in the treatment of skeletal metastases in patients with breast cancer or osteolytic lesions of multiple myeloma: a phase III, double-blind, comparative trial. *Cancer J.* 2001;7:377-387.
32. Berenson JR, Crowley JJ, Grogan TM, et al. Maintenance therapy with alternate-day prednisone improves survival in multiple myeloma patients. *Blood.* 2002;99:3163-3168.
33. Interferon as therapy for multiple myeloma: an individual patient data overview of 24 randomized trials and 4012 patients. The Myeloma Trialists' Collaborative Group. *Br J Haematol.* 2001;113:1020-1034.
34. Richardson PG, Barlogie B, Berenson J, et al. A phase 2 study of bortezomib in relapsed, refractory myeloma. *N Engl J Med.* 2003;348:2609-2617.
35. Richardson PG, Sonneveld P, Schuster MW, et al. Bortezomib or high-dose dexamethasone for relapsed multiple myeloma. *N Engl J Med.* 2005;352:2487-2498.
36. Sipe JD, Cohen AS. Amyloidosis. In: Fauci AS, Braunwald E, Isselbacher KJ, Wilson JD, et al, eds. *Harrison's Principles of Internal Medicine.* 14th ed. New York, NY: McGraw-Hill; 1998:1856-1860.
37. Comenzo RL, Gertz MA. Autologous stem cell transplantation for primary systemic amyloidosis. *Blood.* 2002;99:4276-4282.
38. Skinner M, Sanchorawala V, Seldin DC, et al. High-dose melphalan and autologous stem-cell transplantation in patients with AL amyloidosis: an 8-year study. *Ann Intern Med.* 2004;140:85-93.

Index

Note: Italicized page locators indicate a figure; tables are indicated with a *t*

A

B

C

G

H

I

J

K

L

M

N

Q

R

T

U

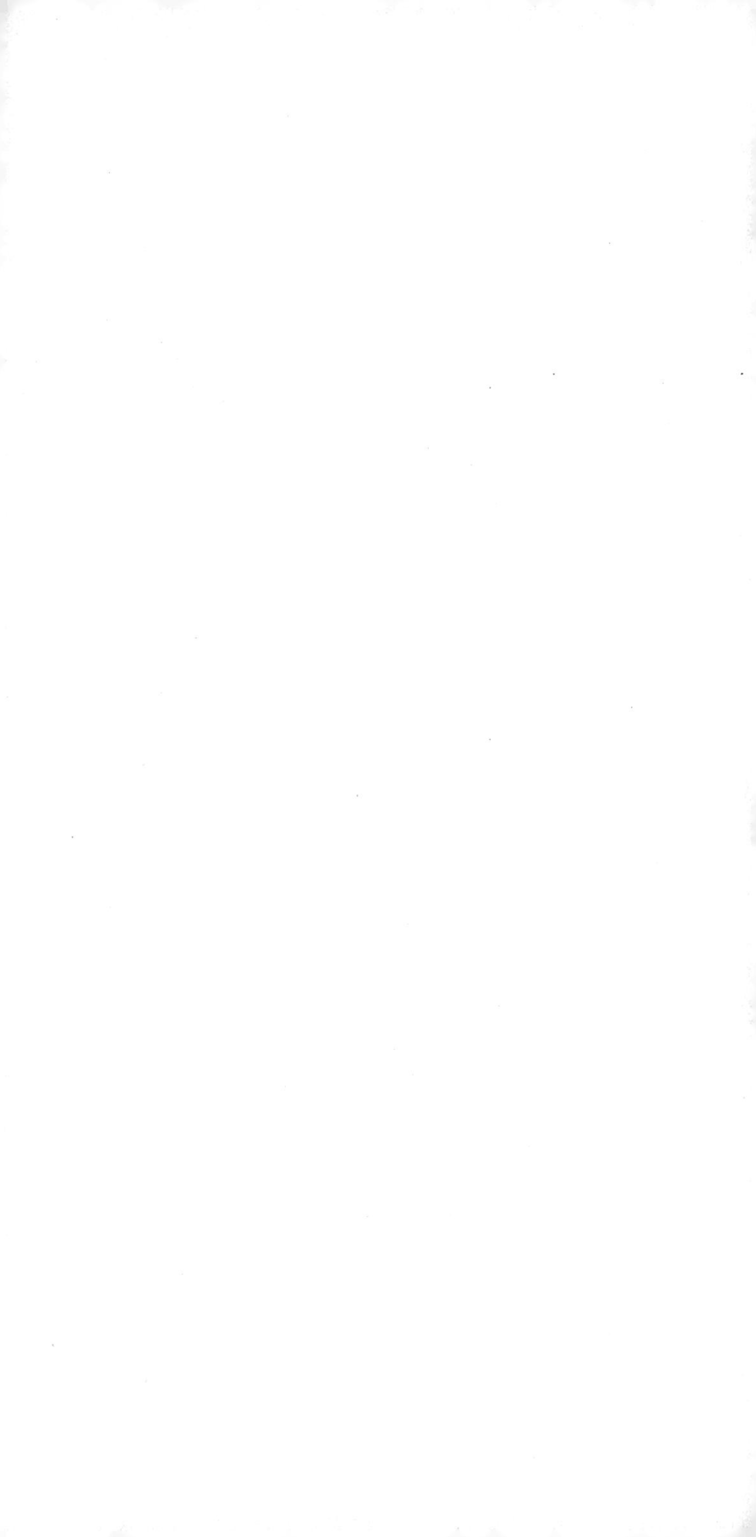

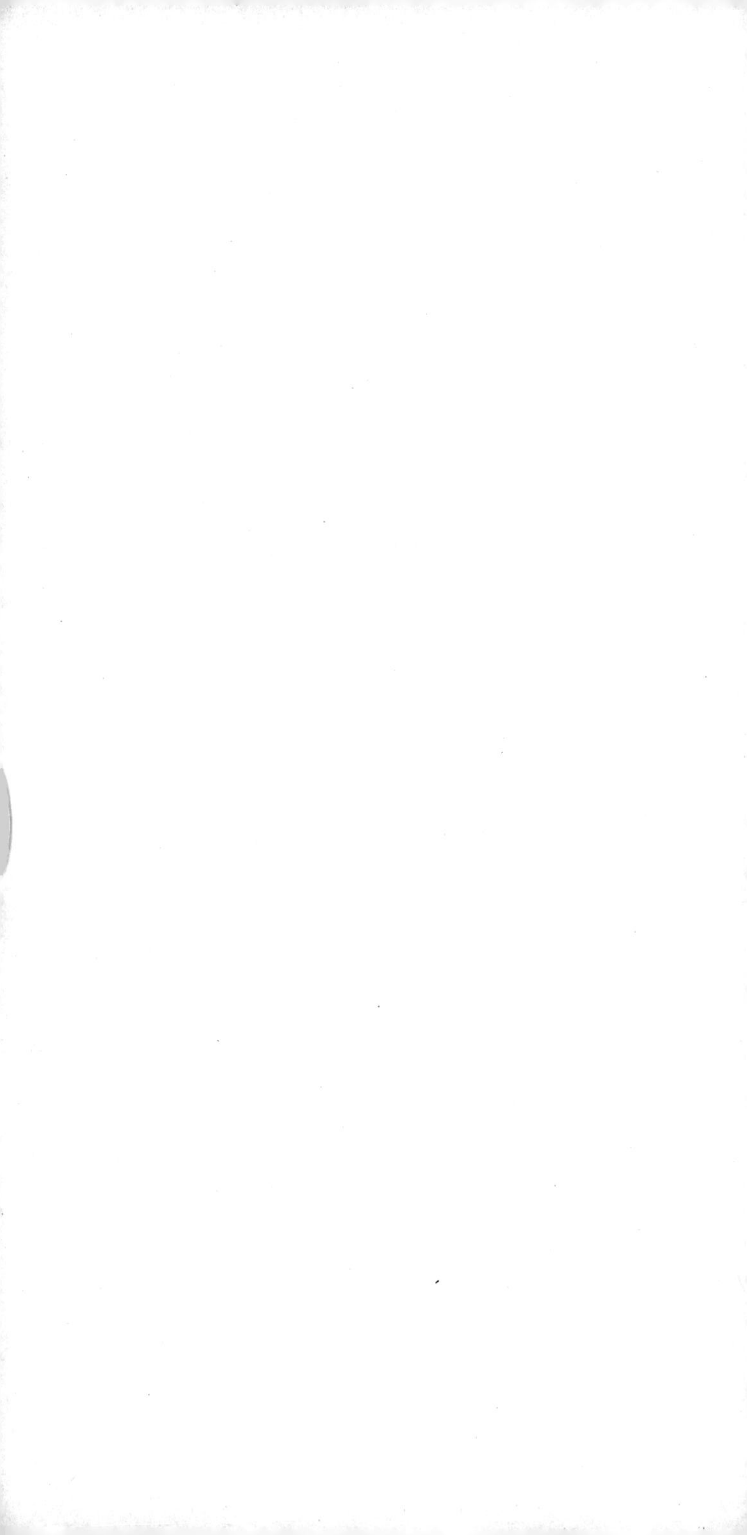